HEART DISEASE:
Questions You Have ... Answers You Need

Other titles in this series:

ARTHRITIS: *Questions You Have ... Answers You Need*
ASTHMA: *Questions You Have ... Answers You Need*
BLOOD PRESSURE: *Questions You Have ... Answers You Need*
DEPRESSION: *Questions You Have ... Answers You Need*
DIABETES: *Questions You Have ... Answers You Need*
HEARING LOSS: *Questions You Have ... Answers You Need*
PROSTATE: *Questions You Have ... Answers You Need*
VITAMINS AND MINERALS: *Questions You Have
... Answers You Need*

By the same author:

BLOOD PRESSURE: *Questions You Have
... Answers You Need*

HEART DISEASE:

Questions You Have ... Answers You Need

Ed Weiner

Consultant editor Dr Robert Youngson

Thorsons
An Imprint of HarperCollinsPublishers

Thorsons
An Imprint of HarperCollins*Publishers*
77–85 Fulham Palace Road,
Hammersmith, London W6 8JB
1160 Battery Street,
San Francisco, California 94111–1213

Published by Thorsons 1997
1 3 5 7 9 10 8 6 4 2

© The People's Medical Society 1985, 1991, 1992, 1997

The People's Medical Society asserts the moral right to
be identified as the author of this work

A catalogue record for this book
is available from the British Library

ISBN 0 7225 3312 8

Printed in Great Britain by
Caledonian Book Manufacturing Ltd, Glasgow

All rights reserved. No part of this publication may be
reproduced, stored in a retrieval system, or transmitted,
in any form or by any means, electronic, mechanical,
photocopying, recording or otherwise, without the prior
permission of the publishers.

CONTENTS

PUBLISHER'S NOTE

No popular medical book, however detailed, can ever be considered a substitute for consultation with, or the advice of, a qualified doctor. You will find much in this book that may be of the greatest importance to your health and wellbeing, but it is not intended to replace your doctor or to discourage you from seeking his or her advice.

If anything in this book leads you to suppose that you may be suffering from the conditions with which it is concerned, you are urged to see your doctor without delay.

Every effort has been made to ensure that the contents of this book reflect current medical opinion and that it is as up to date as possible, but it does not claim to contain the last word on any medical matter.

Terms printed in **boldface** can be found in the glossary, beginning on *page 144*. Only the first mention of the word in the text is emboldened.

INTRODUCTION

Heart disease is the number-one killer of the Western world; in our over-fed and under-exercised society there is more heart disease than any other major disorder. Although happily there has been some slight reduction in the incidence of heart disease in recent years, it is still out on its own at the head of the list of causes of death. Tragically, a high proportion of these deaths could be avoided.

There are several different kinds of heart disease, but one of them in particular, 'coronary artery disease', stands out as the real killer and the principal cause of human distress and disability. This very common disorder, which is present to a varying degree in almost all men and most post-menopausal women, is the cause of angina and heart attacks, and is the condition that kills some 160,000 people every year in Britain. One of the things that this book explains in some detail is exactly what happens in the coronary arteries of people unfortunate enough to be severely affected. This book also explains what we can do to minimize the chances of this happening to us.

The widely-held view that heart disease predominantly affects high-pressure and highly-stressed business- or professional men is wrong. Of course some of these people suffer heart attacks, but it has been clearly shown by a great deal of careful epidemiological research that heart attacks are significantly more common among ordinary people living ordinary, even mundane lives. They are commonest of all in manual and unskilled workers. This is reflected in the fact that the incidence of heart attacks has a strong geographic basis, rising progressively from south to north in the United Kingdom. The reasons for this unexpected finding are now well established, and these, too, are explained in this book.

Another widely-held view is that cancer, especially breast cancer, is the principal cause of death among women. This, too, is false. Far more women die from coronary heart disease than from any other condition. It is true that during their reproductive years, women are well protected against heart disease; but after the menopause they soon catch up and it is not long before the incidence of deaths from heart disease in women equals or surpasses that in men.

These are important issues, and you owe it to yourself to know about them. *Heart Disease: Questions You Have ... Answers You Need* is a compilation of the most commonly asked questions on this vitally important subject, and offers clear, jargon-free answers. The book also contains an account of the latest research from the medical literature.

Reading this book could save your life.

Dr R. M. Youngson, Series Editor
London, 1997

CHAPTER ONE

THE INSIDE STORY

Q   **Let's get down to basics: What is the heart?**

A   Many people, especially those on the other side of the Atlantic, seem to think that the heart is over on the left side of the chest. You will have seen Americans on TV pledging allegiance to their flag with their right hands or hats over their left breasts. In fact, the heart is in the centre of the chest in an area called the **mediastinum**. (You can feel the beat of your heart on the left side because the heart is tilted a bit to the left, and the part furthest left, the apex, is where the beat is perceived to be strongest.)

   The standard description of the average heart is that it is about the size of your fist, weighs less than a pound, is somewhat pear-shaped, is pinkish-grey in colour and doesn't look a bit like the drawings we used to make of hearts when we were children. It is largely made of muscle, and the muscle is known as the **myocardium**. It's hollow and is divided into a left and right side, each with two chambers (an **atrium** above and a **ventricle** below). It's the pump at the centre of your circulatory system, and it's attached to a network of arteries, veins and tiny **capillaries** so profuse that if everything else in your body were to disappear, you would still be immediately recognizable. Your heart is usually good to you, so long as you're good to it. When the two of you fall out, it can mean the end of a beautiful friendship – and your life.

Your heart is a well-protected piece of machinery. It sits snugly within a sac called the **pericardium** inside a hard shell made up of the **sternum,** or breastbone, to the front of it, the rib cage and lungs around it, the diaphragm under it, and the backbone behind it. This is a masterful design for the protection of an important package, one which any engineer would be proud to have designed.

Q   **What, exactly, does the heart do?**
A   To get a better idea of, and feel for, the work your heart does, let's pretend we can shrink down to the size of a single drop of your blood, and then take the journey it makes through your body.

We'll start in the heart itself; more precisely, in the **left ventricle**, where the blood – tingling with oxygen and ready to travel – is propelled by a forceful tightening of the ventricle (a contraction) into the body's primary **artery**, the **aorta**. The force applied to the blood in the aorta, when measured, is what we've come to know as blood pressure. Coursing along the arterial system, we, in company with countless blood cells and dissolved nutrient substances, are transported through progressively smaller arterial branches – the **arterioles** – until we reach the smallest blood vessels of all – the capillaries – in which we are in intimate contact with the body's tissues. There we deliver our parcel of oxygen and a quantity of fuel (mainly glucose) to the eagerly awaiting body cells. The cells need them to stay alive. Then, after we've collected some waste products and carbon dioxide, we continue on, a little blue and winded, and follow the flow through the body's network of **veins**. On the way back we happen to have passed through part of the intestine and then through the liver, where we pick up more nutrients. Finally, we enter the lower of the two great veins – the **superior** and **inferior vena cavae** – which returns us to the heart. If we had been carried up to the head, we would have returned by way of the superior vena cava.

In the heart, the oxygen-deficient blood from the lower and upper parts of the body passes into the **right atrium**. All of it, including us, is then pumped out through the right ventricle into the **pulmonary artery** and off to the lungs. There, the blood gives up the carbon dioxide waste gas (which you breathe out) and sucks up its fill of oxygen (which you breathe in). We then move with the blood from the lungs to the **left atrium**, where it collects, ready to move into the left ventricle, to be pumped out through the aorta to the rest of the body. And this is where we came in.

Over and over, again and again, this cyclical process – the blood moving from the upper reservoir atrium chambers to the lower pumping ventricle chambers, and out and back through 60,000 miles of veins, arteries and capillaries – goes on day in and day out, your heart squeezing an average of 72 times a minute to maintain the circulation of an average volume of 5 litres of blood.

Q **So is it all this oxygen-rich blood pumping through it that keeps the heart healthy?**

A As a matter of fact, it isn't – at least not directly. Despite the huge volume of blood flowing through the heart each day (some 7,000 litres), none of it directly aids the heart muscle in getting the oxygen and sustenance it needs. Like other parts of the body, the heart receives its 'diet' via a system of arteries. These are called the **coronary arteries** – so-called because these arteries and their branches cover the upper part of the heart like a crown (*corona* is the Latin word for a crown). There are two coronary arteries – the right and the left – but the left coronary immediately divides into two main branches, so doctors often talk as if there were *three* coronary arteries. As with the rest of the body's arterial system, the heart's blood supply derives from arteries which come off the aorta, split into smaller arterioles and then into capillaries which feed the muscle. From the muscle, a system of veins returns the deoxygenated blood to the right atrium. So heart blood follows the shortest route of all.

Coronary heart disease, then, is a severe health problem affecting not so much the heart's muscle directly as the flow of the blood through this 'crown' surrounding and feeding the heart.

Q **What are heart valves? Where are they in the heart, and what do they do?**

A The valves are extremely thin, powerful and efficient 'flood gates' made of heart-lining tissue known as **endo-cardium**. This is also the substance which lines the inner walls of the atria and ventricles. The valves act to keep blood flowing in one direction only so that any compression of the system automatically causes the blood to circulate. There are four valves, and in the course of the blood's journey through the heart it meets these valves in this order: as the deoxygenated blood accumulates in the reservoir of the right atrium, it is briefly kept there by the **tricuspid valve** as the right ventricle contracts. When the tricuspid opens up, the blood flows into the right ventricle, and then is pumped through the **pulmonary valve** into the lungs. The now-oxygenated blood returning from the lungs arrives in the left atrium and is kept briefly within that chamber by the closed **mitral valve** as the left ventricle contracts. When the mitral valve opens, the blood flows into the left ventricle and is pumped through the open **aortic valve** into the aorta and off to the rest of the body. The actual rhythm of the heart means that the mitral and tricuspid valves open and close in unison. This causes the 'lub' sound of the heartbeat, as heard through a stethoscope. Then, upon the heart's contraction, the pulmonary and aortic valves open in unison to allow the blood to flow. This causes the 'dub' sound of the heartbeat.

Q **Speaking of the heart rhythm, what makes the heart contract and beat in the first place?**

A It has to do with the heart's built-in conduction system. If that term – conduction – sounds like something out of electrical engineering, that's just about right. In the wall of the right atrium of your heart, so small that only a microscope can pick it out, is something called the **sinus**, or **sinoatrial** (S-A), **node**. In simple terms, this is your heart's natural pacemaker. What happens is that an

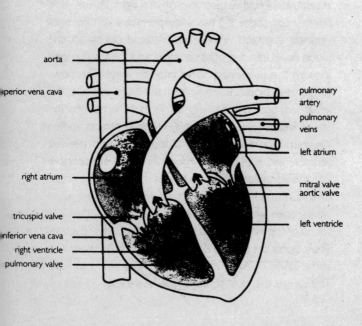

aorta

superior vena cava

pulmonary artery

pulmonary veins

left atrium

right atrium

mitral valve
aortic valve

tricuspid valve

inferior vena cava
right ventricle
pulmonary valve

left ventricle

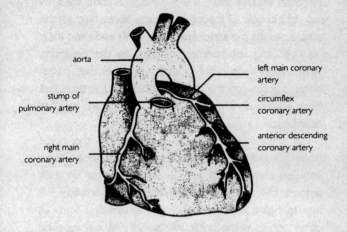

aorta

stump of
pulmonary artery

right main
coronary artery

left main coronary
artery

circumflex
coronary artery

anterior descending
coronary artery

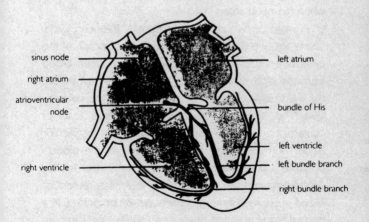

sinus node

right atrium

atrioventricular
node

right ventricle

left atrium

bundle of His

left ventricle

left bundle branch

right bundle branch

electrical impulse from the S-A node is conducted, by way of a bundle of specialized muscle fibres, through the atria, down to the **atrioventricular** (AV) **node** and then, via right and left bundle branches, to the ventricles. When these receive the electrical impulses they immediately tighten (contract). This whole process takes less than a second. The contracting is what we call the heartbeat.

So the heart, unlike other muscles in the body, doesn't need to be stimulated by electrical nerve impulses coming from outside of itself – it can do it all, automatically and with consistency and rhythm. A human heart, even after being disconnected from all other nerves in the body, will, so long as it is supplied with oxygen and fuel, continue to beat about 100 times a minute. The conduction system even has a self-adjusting feature, to alter the force of the contraction when the need arises.

A word or two about the nature of the heart cycle. There are two parts to it: **Diastole** is that portion of the cycle when the heart is at rest – that is, when blood from the atria is pouring into the ventricles, just before the ventricular contraction; the **systole** is the contraction. The two numbers in blood pressure readings correspond to these heartbeat phases, the systolic (or higher number) being a measurement of the blood's pressure against artery walls when the heart is actually contracting, and the diastolic being the measurement of blood pressure during the heart's relaxation period. In a normal blood pressure reading of 120/80 – or '120 over

80' – the systolic pressure is indicated by the 120, the diastolic by the 80. These figures correspond to the pressure exerted by columns of mercury respectively 120 and 80 mm high. So they are said to represent pressure in terms of millimetres of mercury (mm Hg).

Q **How do doctors know if your heart is healthy – or diseased?**

A They find out, mostly, through techniques and tools we're all fairly familiar with.

Best known is the **stethoscope**, invented in the last century by a French doctor called René Théophile Hyacinthe Laënnec (1782–1826). The name 'stethoscope' is hardly appropriate, however, as it comes from Greek roots meaning 'a device for viewing the chest', which, of course, is not what it does. The stethoscope simply allows the doctor conveniently to listen to the goings-on within the chest, transmitting sounds up two flexible plastic tubes to diagnostically discerning ears and brains. An experienced and knowledgeable practitioner can listen to the sounds coming from your chest – which is a rather noisy place, what with all the muscular activity, breathing and so on – and know which are normal and which, such as murmurs, whooshing sounds, crackling or rubbing noises, might be signs of trouble which require further investigation.

During the investigation of the heart, another device a doctor will turn to will be the **sphygmomanometer** (pronounced sfig-mo-mah-NOM-eter). This is the technical name for what most people call a blood pressure machine. A blood pressure reading – whether high, low or just right – will add important information to the diagnostic picture your doctor is forming.

Q **How about electrocardiograms? What do they show?**
A The **electrocardiogram** (ECG) is an amplifying instrument used by doctors either to detect evidence of suspected heart disease or as a routine check in a periodic physical examination. Among the many things an ECG can show well are irregular heartbeat rhythms and signs of heart muscle damage caused by a narrowed or blocked coronary artery.

An electrocardiograph machine picks up the heart's tiny electrical currents through a system of five to 10 electrical leads – metal plates smeared with a wet paste to aid conductivity – placed on a patient's body at locations which have been found best for picking up the heart's electrical impulses: the arms, the legs and various points on the chest. These electrical currents pass through the electrodes and along the insulated leads to the ECG machine. There they are amplified about 3,000 times so as to be able to move a pen and write their specific patterns on a continuously moving strip of graph paper.

Most of us have seen these long, thin black-and-white strips of paper with the heart action scrawled along them in the form of jagged hills and valleys. Here is a typical ECG pattern of waves and spikes, and the alphabetical designations given to each segment:

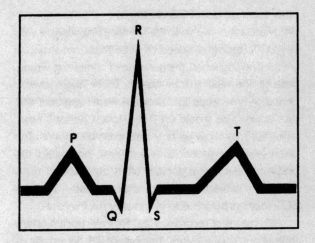

The P wave shows the electrical action within the heart as both atria contract. The Q, R and S waves (called the QRS complex) illustrate what is going on in the ventricles. The T wave shows the ventricles recovering from one contraction and preparing for the next.

Doctors know the normal ECG patterns, and can judge whether what they've just recorded falls within normal ranges or, if not, what the abnormal waves and spikes suggest. Many modern ECG machines automatically analyse the trace, compare it with stored data and suggest a diagnosis. These computerized ECG machines have been shown to give better results than most doctors in the interpretation of the tracings, but do rather less well than expert cardiologists.

Q **How accurate is an ECG reading?**

A Pretty accurate – within limits. For one thing, a single, solitary ECG reading in a doctor's office might not show up anything wrong when there *is* indeed something wrong, because the reading may happen to be taken over a period of time when that problem wasn't apparent and thus couldn't be picked up. Then, too, a person's heart difficulties may show up only after exertion, so a reading taken while the patient is at rest might not detect the problem. That's why doctors often put patients on a treadmill – subjecting them to a **stress test** – and take ECG readings before, during, and after the exercise.

As a means of recording a patient's electrocardiogram throughout daily activities, throughout 24 hours, ambulatory electrocardiographic monitoring (AEM) devices were introduced more than 20 years ago. Since then, these devices have been used for a variety of clinical purposes, including detecting and evaluating irregular heartbeats (called **arrhythmias**); checking on the relationship of symptoms to arrhythmias; estimating the outlook (prognosis) of heart disease; and assessing the effect of anti-arrhythmic and other drugs.

There has, however, been some authoritative criticism of the value of this method. ECGs are not foolproof, they are not good predictors of future heart disease, and they aren't immensely valuable in detecting a number of cardiovascular ills. The ECG is a useful diagnostic tool, but is best used in conjunction with other examinations and tests that will help to confirm a diagnosis.

Q **What are some of these other tests?**

A As the doctor grows more and more certain that a heart disorder – or even a particular heart disorder – is what's troubling you, the tests become more sophisticated and complex, tend to give more information, move into the area of invasive techniques, and carry with them some minor risks.

For example, your doctor might want you to have a chest X-ray to look at heart structures or lung and blood vessel complications, or even might want to inject you with a radioactive dye, or contrast material, which allows the doctor to observe and monitor the function (or malfunction) of the heart's structures. This latter procedure is called **angiography**.

Echocardiography is another diagnostic technique. Ultrasonic waves are aimed at and projected through the chest. These sound waves then strike the heart and its various internal structures and are bounced back. Graphic pictures, or echocardiograms, are made of these ultrasonic echoes, in much the same way as a ship can send sounds into the depths and obtaining an image of the topography of the ocean floor. Echocardiography is a painless procedure which helps the doctor to 'see' problems involving the heart's valves. It is easier and safer than **cardiac catheterization**, although catheterization may be essential to uncover information in certain circumstances.

Q **What is cardiac catheterization?**

A A process in which a thin, flexible tube is inserted in a locally anaesthetized part of the body and then pushed along through a blood vessel (usually in the groin or arm) and on into the heart. To study the right side of the heart, the catheter is snaked through a vein; for the left side, an artery is used. The passage of the catheter tube is observed by doctors using **fluoroscopy**, a specialized X-ray procedure.

When the coronary arteries are being examined, the process is referred to as *coronary arteriography*, while *angiocardiography* is the name for the test when the atria or ventricles are the targets of the probe.

Q   **What is the point of cardiac catheterization?**

A   It is probably the best way yet developed for a doctor to decide if heart surgery is likely to be necessary. The cardiac catheterization process can tell the doctor if the oxygen content of your blood is abnormal, if your cardiac output is low, if there are structural heart defects or valve problems, or how extensive coronary artery disease is and how best surgery can tackle the trouble – if surgery is the answer.

Cardiac catheterization is not a particularly risky procedure, but whenever an invasive technique is used, especially one that involves the heart, there is always some danger. Cardiac catheterization, though useful and relatively painless, should be performed only when absolutely necessary, and should not be taken lightly by either doctor or patient.

CHAPTER TWO

WHEN BAD THINGS HAPPEN TO GOOD HEARTS

Q **What is heart disease? What causes it?**

A This is not an easy question to answer because there is no single entity you can point to and call 'heart disease'. There are many different cardiac and circulatory disorders, with a range of causes involving hereditary or environmental factors, or both. Sometimes there are lots of causes for a single condition, each of them adding to the total picture and the ultimate heart problem. 'Multifactorial' is the term doctors use to describe the causes of these heart diseases. This is the case with the most important one of all – coronary heart disease – as we shall soon see.

If you skim through the medical literature of just the past few years, you'll find that researchers have been ranging far and wide to try and find out whether there is one overwhelmingly important element which has brought about the epidemic of heart disease in the countries of the Western world. Some scientists think heart disease is mainly caused by things we do, others by things we are. Still others think that, to some extent, we are the innocent victims of factors outside our control. This, however, is not a very widely held view.

Q **What do these studies tell us?**

A A lot of them point again and again to the best-known, and what are considered the major, risk factors for those heart diseases which appear to be acquired and avoidable: diets leading to high levels of body choles-terol, smoking, drinking, lack of exercise, stress, obesity, **high blood pressure** – all of which we'll discuss in some length later on.

Beyond these, new reports come out regularly, and some make newspaper headlines. Some underline the obvious, while others break new ground or border on the exotic. Many of them raise more questions than they answer. For example:

- Poverty and heart disease are related. According to one study, heart disease death rates increase as family income declines. What's the reason for this? According to one epidemiologist, less well-to-do people have not profited by good advice to give up bad habits such as smoking, overeating and avoiding exercise, while the better off have modified their behaviour and are more fitness-conscious.
- Sickle cell anaemia may, it is thought, cause heart attacks without any coronary **atherosclerosis** (fatty deposits on coronary artery walls) being involved. Scientists believe that in some black people (that portion of the population which has this condition

almost exclusively) the red blood cells that become sickle-shaped (crescented) during attacks may keep the heart muscle from receiving adequate oxygen supplies, leading to oxygen starvation and ultimately **myocardial infarction** (known most commonly as a heart attack).

- Oestradiol (or oestrogen), a female sex hormone, has been found to be present in higher levels in men who get heart attacks than in men who don't. What this could mean, say researchers, is that coronary heart disease may be primarily a hormonal disorder. Why the high levels of a female hormone show up in some men, how it happens, and what to do about it are puzzling at the moment.

- A number of studies indicate that noise — industrial, environmental, etc. — may lead to high blood pressure and heart problems. People who live near airports or under flight paths, according to some research, tend to have blood pressure abnormalities, higher pulse rates and a number of other cardiovascular changes. And, worst of all, children appear to be most affected by this dangerous noise pollution.

- We know that oestrogens are protective against heart attacks in women. Higher insulin production in women might be another of the reasons why pre-menopausal women generally have lower heart disease mortality and better blood-fat levels than men. It's not known why, exactly. It might have something to do with the way insulin acts as a hypotensive **vasodilator** – that is, as a mechanism for opening the blood vessels wider, allowing blood to flow through more easily and thus reducing the force of the blood pressure. It has also been shown that diabetes tends to equalize the level of heart disease among men and women.

- A small proportion of the hundreds of thousands of sudden cardiac deaths every year may be the result of some kind of allergic reaction. Researchers have found histamine – a chemical produced in the body, especially in the nasal passages and lungs, when the body comes into contact with something it is sensitive to – in human heart muscle, and this release of histamine causes the heartbeat rate to increase twofold. What the scientists are suggesting, in other words, is that while an allergen may affect your nose in a way that causes you to sneeze, your heart during an allergic reaction may respond in the form of sudden cardiac arrest. This is probably not a very significant finding, however.

- There seems to be a positive association between retirement among men and subsequent death from coronary heart disease. According to researchers, the risk of heart disease among men who are retired may be 80 per cent higher than among those who are still working, or who continue to work. Said one of the doctors involved in the study: 'It is possible that we may have stumbled across a new risk factor, because many of those who die of heart attacks have none of the established risk factors, and that's why we are searching for possible psychosocial stress factors, such as retirement.'

- According to another report, men whose height is 5 feet 7 inches and under appear to be up to 70 per cent more likely to have a heart attack than those who are 6 feet 1 inch and above. The results are similar to those from a previous study which found a higher risk of heart attacks in shorter women than in taller ones. The speculation is that smaller people have smaller coronary vessels which are more vulnerable to blockage.

These are just a few of the intriguing points that have been thrown up by medical research. There are many others. As to which, if any, is the principal cause – the real source of heart problems – or if there is, in fact, one outstanding factor, remains to be seen. While in many instances the cause of heart problems is not clear, many of the ways in which heart disease arise are now well understood or are becoming clearer. In the rest of this section we'll define and explore these illnesses, conditions and defects.

CONGENITAL HEART DEFECTS

Q **What are congenital heart defects?**
A They are, as the word **congenital** implies, structural defects or abnormalities that are present at birth due to developmental defects in the foetus, whether genetic or

otherwise. They are, in short, parts of the heart or major blood vessels which have developed incorrectly or incompletely.

Q   **How common are congenital defects?**
A   Very common. Many thousands of babies are born each year with heart defects. At least 35 types of congenital heart defects are recognized.

Q   **Is a congenital defect always a death sentence?**
A   Definitely not. Millions of people with heart defects are alive and well today.

Q   **Why do these congenital defects occur?**
A   Any number of possible reasons, very few of which are completely understood by medical science. German measles (rubella) acquired by the mother early in pregnancy is a well-known cause of defects in some cases. Certain drugs seem to cause birth defects – pregnant women should be extremely careful about taking any kind of medication. And that goes for alcohol, too. Down's syndrome children may have cardiac abnormalities. Other environmental factors may contribute to some defects.

Q   **How obvious are these defects? Are they noticed and taken care of straight away?**
A   By about the age of five, nearly all congenital defects will have shown themselves or been discovered. More than half of these cases are noted during the

baby's first year of life. Severe cases are often fatal very soon after birth. Others may be noted and followed up through the teen years and adult life without any surgery or other treatment being required. Sometimes problems in people in their late years are due to complications of the surgery they had when they were young.

Q **How do doctors know if someone has a congenital defect or not?**

A Severe defects cause a bluish tinge in the skin (*cyanosis*) and may cause breathlessness after only minor effort. Less severe abnormalities may be detected by hearing a murmur, or unusual (out of the ordinary) sound during a routine examination.

Q **Do all murmurs indicate that congenital heart disease is present?**

A No. Some murmurs are what are called 'innocent' murmurs – not dangerous, not indicative of any disease, really – and they often occur naturally in young people and adolescents. A knowledgeable family doctor or specialist can usually tell the difference between innocent murmurs and significant murmurs by identifying the differing hums, clicks and vibrations heard and felt during an examination of the heart and chest area. X-rays and ECGs are also used in the classification, detection, confirmation or negation of suspected significant murmurs.

For more definite and conclusive diagnosis, people

with possibly serious murmurs or newly discovered defects may be asked to undergo cardiac catheterization, but a careful doctor will put off this invasive procedure until after non-invasive echocardiography is performed – and will then only use it if surgery seems to be likely to be necessary to correct the problem. Echocardiography can tell the doctor a lot, and may rule out the need for invasive – and more dangerous – techniques. Ultrasound, **CT scans** (computer-enhanced views of slices of anatomy) and **magnetic resonance imaging** (MRI) are other methods used to get better pictures of the heart.

Q **What do all these tests and machines show the doctor?**

A Quite a lot – everything from valve defects to changes in the heart size (usually enlargement), from blood flow to any abnormalities of the major blood vessels.

Q **What are some of the more common congenital heart defects?**

A One very complex defect is known as the *tetralogy of Fallot*. This is by no means the most common form of congenital heart defect, but is mentioned first because any part of the tetralogy may be present on its own. The word tetralogy indicates that the problem is fourfold, and these are the four:

1 an unnatural opening between the right ventricle and the left ventricle (*ventricular septal defect*)

2 severe narrowing of the pulmonary artery
   (*pulmonary stenosis*)
3 thickening of the muscular wall of the right ventricle
   (*ventricular hypertrophy*)
4 a defect in which the aorta gets blood from both the
   right and the left ventricles, called *dextroposition of
   the aorta*.

A ventricular septal defect (hole in the heart), for
instance, is the most common congenital heart defect in
newborn babies. Similarly, the natural opening in the
foetal heart between the two atria may fail to close at
birth as it should. This is called *atrial septal defect*.
Symptoms may not show up until adulthood, when
surgery can correct it. This natural opening is necessary
during foetal life to allow the blood to bypass the lungs
which are not, of course, being used. It normally closes
off when breathing starts and the pressures on the left
side of the heart increase.

Babies with a severe congenital defect such as
the tetralogy of Fallot often have blue skin. The cyanosis,
or blueness, of those afflicted in this way is due to inadequate oxygenation of the blood, the circulation of
which may partially bypass the lungs. Blood which is
low in oxygen has a purplish-blue colour; well-
oxygenated blood is bright red. Other effects are stun-
ting of growth, clubbed fingers and the coughing up
of blood.

Surgery to correct Fallot's tetralogy is often recommended while the child is still quite young. Some

people may live to adulthood without surgery, and live near-normal lives – but they risk later complications including brain abscesses and infections of the heart. In some severe cases, however, surgery is, unfortunately, impossible.

In *patent ductus arteriosus*, the passage between the aorta and the pulmonary artery (the ductus arteriosus) – which remains open in the foetus until the time of birth – fails to close up. The symptoms don't show up, usually, until the child is older, and then stunted growth and breathing difficulties become apparent. Surgery can shut the opening and, if performed early enough (before the child reaches the teen years), the results may be excellent.

Coarctation of the aorta is a severe congenital narrowing of this major vessel. This can cause really high blood pressure in the upper part of the body, especially during exercise, because the normal, forceful thrust of blood from the heart meets tremendous resistance when it tries to pass though the narrowed portion of the misshapen aorta. The blood pressure in the lower part of the body is well below normal.

Another condition that causes cyanosis is *Eisenmenger's syndrome*, another type of ventricular septal defect with additional complications.

HEART VALVE DISEASE

Q **What is valvular heart disease?**

A To understand this you first have to have quite a good idea of what the valves look like and what they do.

The valves, as we've noted before, stand like sentries all along the path of the blood as it passes through and out of the heart. Healthy valves, when open, allow blood to move in the proper forward direction; when closed, they prevent the blood from streaming backwards. The valves' unique construction – separate thin leaves which flap open to form a mouth to let the flow through, then flap together and shut tight like lips – acts to prevent any backwash (**valvular regurgitation**).

Certain diseases or conditions damage the valves. For instance, **rheumatic fever** leads to **endocarditis**. This is an inflammation of the heart's inner lining which commonly affects the valves, causing inflammation. As they heal, the valves' flaps develop scar tissue, and this causes them to become distorted and prevents them from closing tightly together. Blood can then leak through the gnarled opening either backwards (regurgitation) or forwards when the valve ought to be closed. In severe cases, as much as 50 per cent of the ejected blood may pass in the wrong direction. Doctors often hear this as a murmur. The scarring can also lead to a narrowing (or *stenosis*) of the valve opening. This condition worsens, and usually requires surgery to repair or replace the valve.

Another way the valve leaves become damaged is through thickening or the deposition of chalk (*calcification*). And there are a number of additional, non-rheumatic valve disorders: floppy valve syndrome (which is rather what it sounds like), syphilitic heart disease, certain tumours, and drug-induced valvular difficulties, among others.

In valve defects, the heart chambers need to work harder to keep up the proper pumping pressure despite the narrowings and the leaks, and this frequently leads to serious complications affecting the size of the ventricles, the thickness of the ventricle walls, and general overwork of the pumping mechanism. In severe cases the heart may simply be unable to maintain an adequate circulation of the blood.

Q   **How do doctors determine for sure that what a patient has is heart disease?**

A   The usual assortment of technological steps, which should move up the ladder from non-invasive (stethoscope, fluoroscopic X-ray, echocardiography) to invasive (cardiac catheterization, angiography). Most experts agree that the most conclusive kind of information about the extent of valve damage and all its complications comes from cardiac catheterization and angiography.

Q   **What kind of surgery can I expect if I have valve troubles?**

A   It would depend on the nature of the problem and its extent.

There is a procedure called **commissurotomy**, in which valve leaves – stuck together because of the scar tissue formed after a bout of rheumatic fever-induced endocarditis – are separated. This procedure doesn't always have to be done as open-heart surgery – during which the heart is stopped and blood flow is detoured through a heart-lung machine – but sometimes can be done while the heart continues its work. In commissurotomy, either a special tool or simply the surgeon's finger is used to separate the scar-sealed leaves.

Another operation, called **annuloplasty**, is sometimes suggested. In this, the surgeon actually reconstructs the valve tissue in a kind of plastic surgery technique.

Unfortunately, in some cases the leaves are in very poor shape, or they go back to sticking to each other again. That's when further surgery – usually valve replacement – is called for.

Q How safe is valve replacement surgery?
A Within limits, it's safe. But any operation has its risks – especially when concerned with the heart. Possible complications, in addition to those associated with any operation, include the danger of rejection of biological valves.

Q Tell me more about these complications.
A Every operation carries some degree of risk – from the anaesthetic, from accidents during surgery, from unexpected bleeding or excessive blood loss, even, in this case, from cardiac arrest. These risks are, fortunately,

very slight nowadays. Modern anaesthesia is particularly safe, and anaesthetists go to great pains to ensure an adequate oxygen supply at all times. The loss of a full oxygen supply is the major danger during surgery, and most anaesthetists now monitor the blood levels of oxygen continuously by means of a device known as a *pulse oximeter*.

The replacement valves inserted into the heart to do the job of diseased mitral or aortic valves are in one way or another fashioned by human hands. Some – called prosthetic valves – are entirely synthetic, made of plastics, metal and other moulded and shaped products. These last quite a while, but may fail. An alternative is an aortic valve taken from a pig, or valves made of other tissue, attached to a ring or skin graft mould.

There are possible problems and complications associated with both of these options. The plastic type sometimes encourages blood clotting – that is, it creates a **thromboembolism** (floating blood clot) which moves in the bloodstream until it reaches and blocks up a narrow blood vessel. This can be really serious, and blood clots of this sort showing up in the wrong place can lead to life-threatening crises. Recipients of artificial valves are often prescribed anti-clotting (anticoagulant) drugs to try to prevent this problem.

Other complications include separation of the ring from where it is attached to the heart, infection and – in tissue replacement valves – deterioration or calcification similar to what happened to the original valves, sometimes within 10 to 15 years of implant. Frequently, valve difficulties show up in a heart that is also suffering from coronary artery disease, which brings its own complications, as we'll soon see. Your surgeon may have to consider whether he or she should perform coronary artery bypass surgery at the same time as putting in a new valve. A discussion of bypass surgery and other alternatives can be found later in this book.

The type of surgery needed, the type of valve, if replacement is necessary, the need for simultaneous bypass surgery and the risks and complications involved should all be discussed with the surgeon before a decision is made and consent given.

Q Any other complications?

A A few postoperative ones, especially the danger of endocarditis. Infection is a tremendous threat to the re-valved heart, and thus other operations, including dental surgery, should be accompanied by careful and sufficient antibiotic treatment. Dentistry is commonly associated with a transient passage into the blood of certain germs (*streptococci*) that are normally found in the mouth. These germs are harmless to healthy people, but in people liable to endocarditis they can be very dangerous and can cause accumulations of loose material called *vegetations* on the valves. This condition, known as *bacterial endocarditis*, was once nearly always fatal before the advent of antibiotics.

Drugs to prevent blood clotting (anticoagulants), which will probably have to be taken for life in those with prosthetic valves, can be worrying – especially so in women who become pregnant. They may cause miscarriages or birth defects. That's why women of childbearing age who need heart valve replacement might be wise to opt for the tissue-type valve implant, which may not require accompanying anticoagulant therapy.

HEARTBEAT IRREGULARITIES

Q   **What are heartbeat irregularities?**

A   During attacks of irregular heartbeat, the beats, instead of being even in rhythm and force, become irregularly spaced and variable in strength. They may also speed up or slow down. This can be frightening when it occurs suddenly, or even if it is a frequent event, because that critical organ inside you which has always been faithful, quiet and true now seems to have a wild, misfiring mind of it own. And you feel as if you can't do a thing about it.

Conditions of abnormal heartbeat and rhythm, known generally as arrhythmias, have a multitude of causes, may take a wide variety of forms and, luckily, have a fairly well-established set of responses for controlling or eliminating them.

Some of the things that set off arrhythmias are:

• a diminished amount of oxygen reaching the heart muscle (**hypoxia**) from a blockage which causes a reduced or completely absent flow of coronary

blood (**ischaemia**)
- an unnaturally slow heartbeat (**bradycardia**)
- certain kinds of drugs
- other changes in the physical, electrical or chemical properties of the heart.

Sometimes arrhythmias occur in people with heart disease who are taking the medication **digitalis,** especially if too much is being taken so that digitalis toxicity is present or if the person is potassium-deficient. This is a possible side-effect of having taken **diuretics.** Arrhythmias may also arise from magnesium deficiency or an excess of calcium in the blood.

Q   **Are all arrhythmias life-threatening?**

A   No. Nearly all of us have had an arrhythmic episode at one time or another. That's when, for no apparent reason, we feel an odd 'flip-flop' in our heart, or feel as if our heart has just stopped for a second. Most hearts do that every once in a while, and it usually doesn't mean much. Drugs or other therapy are probably not required, unless these events persist and cause disability, or signify real heart trouble.

Even some of the more serious arrhythmias aren't of grave concern in themselves, although they may be signs that a worrying heart condition is present or that some other physical problems exist.

Q   **For example?**

A   Well, for example, there is **sinus bradycardia**. This is a very slow heartbeat, of 60 beats per minute or less when the heart is at rest. Sometimes, as in fit athletes, this is simply a normal, and enviable, state of affairs, but it may also be a sign of disorders such as underactivity of the thyroid gland (**hypothyroidism**) and abnormally low body temperature (**hypothermia**), to name just two. And certain prescribed drugs, especially tranquillizers, may also cause the heart to beat very slowly.

A more violent type of attack takes place during **atrial paroxysmal tachycardia**, which is almost the opposite of bradycardia. Here, the heart (actually, the atria) suddenly starts to beat up to 220 times a minute, and just as suddenly returns to normal. The accelerated heartbeat is, curiously, not wild and out of control but absolutely regular – just super-fast. These **tachycardias** happen to people with perfectly normal hearts as well as to those who have congenital defects. The attacks are usually not dangerous or life-threatening, unless some sort of heart disease is also present. You should, however, certainly report any such event to your doctor, though normally recurrences need not require medical attention. Dipping your face into cold water will often end the attack – but if the condition persists, drugs or electrical therapy may be necessary.

A few of the most common of the many types of arrhythmias that respond to therapy are **atrial flutter, atrial fibrillation, sick sinus-node syndrome**, and **heart block**.

Q **Which is the most serious of the arrhythmias?**

A A kind called **ventricular fibrillation**. In this cardiac arrhythmia, the ventricle muscle contracts rapidly but so feebly that the aortic valve refuses to open, and blood stops being pumped. Ventricular fibrillation often happens early in a heart attack. It is divided into a primary phase, during which immediate therapy may save a life, and a secondary phase, which is the sign of the end. Ventricular fibrillation is a form of cardiac arrest.

Q **How are arrhythmias treated?**

A In a number of ways, including drugs, electrical stimulation and physical external resuscitation. They are used in different ways for different types of arrhythmia.

Q **Could you explain how these work?**

A Let's take medications first. There are a number of drugs that can calm down the arrhythmic heart, usually by directly affecting the heart's electrical conduction system. One of the better known and most often prescribed drugs for arrhythmia is quinidine (a relative of the antimalarial drug quinine). Quinidine is used in cases of rapid arrhythmias in both the atria and ventricles. Other drugs used for this purpose include:

- lidocaine (a local anaesthetic used to control ventricular arrhythmias)
- propranolol, a **beta-blocker**, used for atrial flutter or fibrillation and also when stress causes arrhythmias, when digitalis toxicity leads to

ventricular arrhythmias, and in cases of heart attack
• procainamide.

Each of these drugs does something different in its own way, and each has a list of side-effects including gastrointestinal disorders, rashes and occasionally more serious complications. These are potent drugs whose use and dosage have to be precise.

Q You mentioned electrical stimulation as a technique used against arrhythmias. What kind of electrical stimulation? How does it work?

A Since the disturbances in the heart which cause arrhythmias are electrical in origin, they can be set right by an electric shock or by providing artificial regular electrical stimuli.

The first way electricity is used to fight arrhythmias is in the case of life-threatening ventricular fibrillations. The piece of technology involved is called a **defibrillator**, and it's basically two metal paddles connected to a source of high-voltage electricity. When a person goes into ventricular fibrillation these paddles – held by a qualified professional who is very well grounded and insulated – are placed on the person's chest.

Through these paddles and into the body passes a jolt so powerful that it actually throws the switch on the heart's electrical impulses and cuts off the current, so to speak. Then, hopefully, the heart's natural pacemaker steps in, regains control over the heartbeat, and gets things back to normal. **Defibrillation** will usually have to be supplemented by artificial ventilation – often by mouth-to-mouth respiration, external cardiac compression, and the administration of drugs and fluids all at the same time.

Defibrillation does not always work, and even when it does the effects don't always last. People in ventricular fibrillation who are shocked back to regular heartbeat are obviously people with sick hearts, and may at any time start fibrillating again. They have to be watched very carefully.

There are no important side-effects to defibrillation. Burnt skin caused by the voltage is a small price to pay for saving a life. If brain damage occurs this is not the result of defibrillation but of its failure to restart the heart soon enough or of undue delay in applying it.

Q **Is there any other way electrical stimulation helps people with arrhythmias?**

A There is a good deal of interest in relatively new devices called automatic defibrillators, which are available in any hospital. These little boxes are attached to the heart of people who have had or continue to have episodes of ventricular fibrillation. The automatic implantable defibrillator actually senses when fibrillation is about to happen and gives off a pulse of electric current which stops it before it gets going.

This device may become a widespread and popular lifesaving tool. Until that time, the most important electrical stimulation mechanism used to fight arrhythmias remains the artificial pacemaker.

Q **How do pacemakers work?**

A Pacemakers are tiny, lightweight mechanisms placed in the chest (although temporary pacemakers are usually not implanted) that give off a rhythmical electrical signal capable of prompting the heart into contraction. This pulsed signal takes over the job of the heart's own faulty natural pacemaker and keeps the heartbeat regular. The spikes of current are generated by an electronic oscillator fed by long-lasting batteries in the pacemaker, and are carried to the heart via an insulated wire at the end of which is a bare electrode. The electrode is placed at the right ventricle during a procedure which takes about 30 to 90 minutes (although a hospital stay could be involved).

The pace of the desired beat may be adjusted at a fixed rate by the cardiologist or other medical personnel. Many pacemakers work 'on demand', taking over only when conditions require them to do so; this lets the heart's own natural pacemaker stay on the job when and for as long as it can. Modern, miniaturized electronic circuits allow a reduction in the size of pacemakers (they are about the size of a rather thick 50p piece, and weigh about 2 ounces) and an increased range of action. In fact, in some pacemakers the rate of firing and various adjustments to the electrical pulses produced can be adjusted by radio, as required. They can also be hooked up to a telephone or Internet computer and readings can be sent via phone lines to monitoring equipment in a hospital clinic.

The two most important conditions which call for a

pacemaker are: complete heart block – in which the heart's own electrical transmission reaches the atria but is not conducted to the ventricles, thus causing the atria and ventricles to beat at different rates – and sinus node difficulties.

Pacemakers are marvels of medical technology, keeping people alive who just a few years ago would have died. But they, and the way they operate, are not without drawbacks and controversy.

Q   **What are these drawbacks? Are they serious?**

A   As we become more and more sophisticated in the realm of technology, mechanical complications and failures are becoming rarer. Still, more often than anybody would like, there are unfortunate events when pacemakers go wrong because of mechanical flaws, sudden battery drain, detached electrodes or broken wires. Occasionally a pacemaker goes haywire and actually creates arrhythmias. Sometimes the ventricle is accidentally punctured by the pacemaker leads, sometimes (as with any implanted device) infection and other problems occur.

Luckily, since the procedure is a relatively common one, there is a lot of expertise and information about implanting and repairing pacemakers, and really serious troubles are infrequent.

Q   **Earlier you mentioned external resuscitation?**

A   The method used – keeping the heart and lungs operating during cardiac arrest by physically pressing against the heart and breathing into the lungs – is called **cardiopulmonary resuscitation**, or **CPR**. It is a widely used lifesaver which anybody can do and everybody should know about.

HEART MUSCLE DISEASES

Q **What can go wrong with the heart muscle itself?**

A Quite a lot, unfortunately. Heart muscle disease – **cardiomyopathy**, to use the proper medical terminology – affects that part of the heart which provides the force of the pumping action – the thick, muscular walls of the ventricles. In cardiomyopathies, and there are several types, the heart walls may increase abnormally in thickness, become rigid and inflexible, shrink to smaller than normal size or thin and balloon out to a disproportionate size. Each of these abnormalities causes a serious problem, including **congestive heart failure**, reduced cardiac output and valvular regurgitation, to name just three.

Q **Why and how does the heart muscle become diseased?**

A In some cases infections are responsible; in others nutritional deficiencies are to blame. Various illnesses and disorders of tissue growth or breakdown (*metabolic upsets*) can lead to cardiomyopathies. Degenerative diseases of the muscles, such as muscular dystrophy, may affect the heart as well. High blood pressure is also among the hazards, because by overexerting the heart muscle it builds up a bulky, rigid left ventricle, and that can lead to serious heart failure.

Toxic substances are prime offenders, too. And by toxic substances we mean a large number of chemicals and even drugs that are taken in excessive doses. These include such different items as carbon tetrachloride and anti-cancer chemotherapy drugs. But the most frequent chemical cause of cardiomyopathy is alcohol, when taken in excess.

Probably the most common cause of cardiomyopathy is repeated small episodes of damage to the muscle from what are really mini-heart attacks. These may occur, as we shall see later, without symptoms – but the cumulative effect may be very serious. It has to be said that many cardiologists do not include this process in the list of causes of cardiomyopathy. All of them agree that this happens, and that it happens quite often, but they think that this process should be classified with coronary heart disease rather than with cardiomyopathy. This is really an academic argument, however, and one that need not concern us here.

With the exception of the latter, all the causes we have mentioned account for only a small proportion of cases of cardiomyopathy. The fact is that nobody knows what causes most cases. Just to confuse you completely, it has to be said that quite a few cardiologists insist that cardiomyopathies are those disorders of heart muscle for which a cause cannot be found.

Q **What are the symptoms of cardiomyopathy?**

A These vary from case to case, but most feature fainting (known as **syncope**), angina and, above all, breathlessness. A great many cases of cardiomyopathy end in heart failure (see below) because, although the ventricles may be enlarged they invariably have seriously diminished pumping power. In addition, the arrhythmia known as atrial fibrillation, in which the pulse is irregular in force and rhythm, is a common symptom of cardiomyopathy. The pulse may be jerky and there may be characteristic murmurs which can be heard with a stethoscope.

Q **How is cardiomyopathy treated?**

A Again it's a matter of selecting the best strategies to tackle the most pressing effects. In cardiomyopathies that lead to heart failure, it is the latter that has to be treated, by using salt reduction, diuretics and high blood pressure-reducing drugs. In some other types of cardiomyopathy, especially when an anatomical obstruction is the problem, surgery is usually the right approach. In some instances, unfortunately, neither medicine nor surgery can help. In these cases, where a disease has widely infiltrated and damaged the heart muscle irreparably, death by heart failure or heartbeat disorders is the usual end result.

PERICARDIAL DISEASE

Q **What's this all about?**

A The pericardium is the sac the heart sits in. This sac is double-walled and secretes a thin film of lubricating fluid between the layers so that they can move smoothly one over the other as the heart beats. The pericardium, like all the other parts of the heart, is prone to diseases of its own, and may be an indicator of infections and/or diseases elsewhere in the body which have travelled to the heart and set up an inflammation, causing one or other of the forms of **pericarditis**.

Q **What are some of the most common types of pericarditis? How are they treated?**

A Probably the most common cause of **acute pericarditis** is damage to the underlying muscle, which occurs in a heart attack. In these cases, however, attention is directed more specifically to the life-threatening attack on the heart muscle; the pericarditis is considered incidental. Other cases are due to one of a number of general diseases (see below). **Acute nonspecific pericarditis** is a condition in which the pericarditis is not secondary to another known disease, but rather is attacked directly itself by a virus.

Whatever the cause, the affected pericardium causes chest pain, fever, and the sound (heard through a stethoscope) of dry (frictionless) rubbing in the sac, synchronous with the heartbeat. ECGs also show irregularities characteristic of acute pericarditis. The treatment of acute pericarditis is the treatment of the underlying causes. These need to be managed before the pericardial infection can be eliminated. Acute nonspecific pericarditis and bacterial infective pericarditis are treated by controlling the infections that cause them with antibiotics and, when viruses are involved for which there is no specific treatment, by controlling the inflammation with anti-inflammatory drugs such as indomethacin.

Pericardial effusion is the name of a condition in which the pericardium becomes flooded with liquid. The liquid, or effusion, arises because the inflamed sac secretes far too much of the normal fluid and may also produce pus and other inflammatory discharge. The damage to the pericardium may come from:

- certain drugs (e.g. minoxidil, an antihypertensive drug)
- certain cancers
- radiation therapy used to fight cancers
- previous heart surgery
- kidney failure requiring immediate dialysis (*uraemia*)
- sarcoidosis
- severe bacterial infection elsewhere in the body
- connective tissue diseases such as systemic lupus erythematosus.

Too much fluid in the pericardium can actually squeeze and compress the heart, getting in the way of the heart's filling up with blood; this is called **cardiac tamponade**. Pericardial effusion can be treated by passing a needle into the sac to drain off the excess fluid. This is called **paracentesis**, or pericardial tap.

A number of the conditions responsible for acute pericarditis and pericardial effusion – kidney failure, exposure to radiation, and tuberculosis, to name a few – may lead to another, quite serious problem called **constrictive pericarditis**. In this, the sac becomes scarred and hard and full of calcium deposits. The heart is no longer free to move about and its ability to contract and dilate is interfered with. In essence, the heart becomes a prisoner, caught in a rigid web that used to be its soft, flexible cushion. Surgical removal of the pericardium is necessary to set things right, although this is a potentially dangerous procedure.

Besides these pericardial problems there are others that are more rare, including tumours and congenital defects.

Now we come to the most important class of all heart disorders – those caused by an inadequate blood supply to the heart muscle.

ISCHAEMIC HEART DISEASE AND ANGINA

Q **What does 'ischaemic heart disease' mean, exactly?**
A Well, ischaemia means that because an artery has become either narrower than normal or blocked up

altogether, there is a deficiency or total absence of blood (and thus oxygen) supply. When this narrowing or blockage occurs in the coronary arteries, it's known as ischaemic heart disease. When doctors refer to ischaemic heart disease they are usually speaking of **angina pectoris** and myocardial infarction.

Q **I've heard of angina attacks, and I know many people suffer greatly from them. What are they? What happens during an angina attack?**

A When the coronary arteries are closed by 50 per cent or more, the stage is set for angina. **Plaques** of fatty material and degenerate muscle cell deposits called **atheroma** occur on the artery walls – the main feature of the disease atherosclerosis, the most prevalent form of arterial disease in the Western world. Atherosclerosis accounts for about 90 per cent of cases of angina. Stenosis, or actual narrowing of the arteries themselves, other than by atherosclerosis, is a frequent precursor to angina. Rheumatoid arthritis, systemic lupus erythematosus and other diseases may also have a secondary effect on the coronary arteries so as to narrow them and interfere with normal blood flow. All these, plus spontaneous coronary artery spasms, contribute to the reduced blood flow that causes angina attacks. Note that angina is not a disease but a *symptom* of an underlying arterial heart disease.

What happens is this: during physical exertion, stress or an emotionally-charged situation, in cold weather, or after a big meal, the heart beats faster and requires more oxygenated blood flow to the muscle to maintain the muscular contractions. But if the channels by which the blood and oxygen flow to the heart are narrowed, not enough nutrients get to the heart muscle tissue. It suffers oxygen deficiency, and the result is the pain of angina pectoris.

This pain can vary considerably from a minor sense of constriction in the chest to a heavy, strangulating, suffocating experience more intense than anything indigestion, chest wall injuries, **pleurisy** or spasms of the oesophagus may cause. Typically, the pain starts under the breastbone, on the left side of the chest, and is of a gripping character. Often it is described as 'having a steel band round the chest'. Commonly the pain radiates out to other places: the left arm, throat, neck, jaw, left shoulder, and occasionally on to the right side. It is an intense, frightening episode. Fortunately, with rest and calm, angina attacks settle completely within a few minutes. If they do not, these symptoms indicate a heart attack and this calls for urgent hospitalization.

Q **How can the doctor tell if what I have is angina pectoris and heart disease or something else that behaves similarly?**

A Most anginal attacks are unmistakable, but not all. Sometimes non-cardiac conditions may cause pain that mimics or comes close to feeling like angina. To determine what's what, the doctor will revert to the usual set of diagnostic tools.

Q **How is angina treated?**

A Behaviourally, medically, and/or surgically.

A change in behaviour – trying to keep calm and handling emotions better and more productively – can work towards limiting the recurrence of anginal episodes. Of course, this just makes attacks less frequent; it doesn't do anything to treat the underlying physical causes of the heart pains.

In a way, this can be said for medication, too. The drugs now available for use in treating angina don't permanently open up the narrowed areas and make things right again. Instead, they temporarily increase the blood flow in the arteries and ease the heart's work. They do this by working to reduce blood pressure, widening the blood vessels and slowing down the heart rate to reduce the heart muscle's oxygen requirements.

Calcium channel blockers are effective drugs used to relieve angina symptoms in those people who suffer attacks even while at rest, when lying down or slee- ping as well as at other times. Some better known and frequently prescribed calcium channel blockers are verapamil (Cordilox, Securon), diltiazem (Adizem, Slozem) and nifedipine (Adilat, Calcilat, Coracten). Each has its side-effects – dizziness and headaches, for example.

Use of thiazide types of blood pressure-lowering medication (diuretics) and digitalis, when heart failure is a factor, are two other drug regimens used to combat angina.

The classic treatment for angina, however, is nitro-glycerin or other drugs in the nitrate family – such as isosorbide (Isordil, Cedocard Retard) or pentaerythritol tetranitrate (Mycardol). These nitrates act as highly effective artery wideners (vasodilators). They are taken in lots of different ways: sometimes they are swallowed; occasionally they're injected intravenously. But more usually they are placed under the tongue so that the drug is absorbed directly from the mouth. A nitroglyc-erin spray is also available, to be sprayed under the tongue during an attack.

Nowadays an even more effective method is commonly used. A patch containing a day's dose of nitroglycerin is placed on the skin, and the nitroglycerin is dispensed transdermally – that is, it passes directly through the skin into the bloodstream. These transder-mal slow-release patches are being used more and more as a way to keep angina attacks from happening, and are far more practical than under-the-tongue nitrate pills. For one thing, there's no fumbling for nitro tablets while in the throes of an attack. Further, the patches last 24 hours; a nitroglycerin pill is good for relieving angina pain, but only for about half an hour or so.

It is common for doctors to prescribe nitrates and calcium channel blockers at the same time, because they help each other out.

Q And what about surgery?

A The surgical route is coronary artery bypass grafting

– commonly known simply as bypass surgery.

We'll be getting to that, and the alternatives to bypass, in a moment. But first let's take a good, hard look at heart attacks.

HEART ATTACK

Q **What exactly *is* a heart attack?**

A Strictly speaking, it's rather less an attack and more a siege.

A blood clot (thrombosis) forms on top of a plaque of atheroma in the lining of a coronary artery and causes an occlusion, or blockage, of that artery. Blood full of oxygen destined for the heart muscle, or myocardium, is blocked off before delivery. What you have is a siege leading to starvation of that portion of the heart muscle which is normally supplied by the closed-off coronary artery branch. As a result, this section of the heart muscle, which is usually in the left ventricle, dies or is severely damaged. Doctors refer to an area of tissue affected in this way as an infarction. Because the infarction occurs in the heart muscle (myocardium) the official medical term for a heart attack is a myocardial infarction. This is commonly abbreviated to MI.

Q **Can you tell me more about how these coronary blockages come about?**

A Atherosclerotic plaques, by themselves, will rarely if ever be large enough to block off a coronary artery branch.

Unfortunately, atheroma interferes with the normal smooth, non-stick property of the arterial lining in the coronary arteries, and small cell fragments in the blood, called platelets, easily adhere to the roughened plaque surface. Platelets crowding and sticking together (aggregation) mean that there is a strong probability that a blood clot will form. This, of course, should never happen within an intact blood vessel. If it happens in a coronary artery branch, the chances are that the clot will quickly increase in size until it has completely closed off the vessel.

The risk of heart attack death by coronary occlusion depends on the size of the branch that is blocked. Occlusion of a whole coronary artery would almost certainly be immediately fatal. Occlusion of a small branch might affect only a very small part of the heart muscle. It is in the cases in between in which the outlook becomes uncertain.

Q How can I tell if I'm having a heart attack?

A You'll know. There's nothing quite like a heart attack. A powerful, crushing, breathtaking pain hits the chest and seems to flow out to the left arm, back, shoulder and throat. There is often an acute and terrifying conviction that you are about to die. The face becomes pale and is doused in a cold, clammy sweat. There is occasionally vomiting – that's why some people at first think that they're merely having a bout of bad indigestion. Many people, in pain and full of panic (which just makes things worse), pass out. Many never regain consciousness – too much heart muscle damage has been caused by an occlusion in a major artery branch.

For angina sufferers, heart attack pain may initially seem like just another, although unusually severe, episode of angina. But when nitroglycerin has no effect and the attack goes on beyond the usual recovery time – in fact, for hours – it's time to get urgent medical assistance. Many people, not believing or willing to face the idea that they are having a heart attack, wait as long as three hours or more before getting help. Delay of this kind could be fatal. If the pain persists for longer than 10 minutes, dial 999, ask for an ambulance and say HEART ATTACK.

That's how *you* can tell if you're having a heart attack. The way doctors tell is by observing the all-too-familiar signs, through ECG readings that indicate disturbance and damage, and through blood tests that measure the change in levels of certain key enzymes which are released by the dying heart muscle cells.

Q Does a person's age or gender put him or her at greater risk of a heart attack?

A Based on the famous Framingham Heart Study, 5 per cent of all heart attacks occur in people under age 40, and 45 per cent occur in people under age 65. In general, coronary heart disease rates are higher for males than for females. Before the menopause, women have considerable protection against heart attacks, apparently because of their oestrogen levels. After the menopause they quickly catch up with men in terms of heart attack risk.

Recent research has added a further twist to the gender question: in what is claimed to be the largest study ever to compare men and women's heart attacks, researchers report that women who have heart attacks are 1.5 times more likely than men to die in hospital, and 1.3 times more apt to die within a year. 'Doctors have long considered heart disease milder in women than in men,' said the study's author, 'but this research shows that doctors must take women's heart symptoms very seriously.'

Another recent study took a similar look at the broader issue of sex differences in the management of coronary artery disease. As reported in the July 25, 1991 issue of the *New England Journal of Medicine*, researchers concluded that despite the fact that coronary artery disease is the leading cause of death in women, 'doctors pursue a less aggressive management approach to coronary disease in women than in men, despite greater cardiac disability in women.'

Q **What is a 'silent heart attack'?**
A It's just that – silent, undetected. It is believed that about one-quarter of all heart attacks are not recognized when they occur. Many people have such 'silent attacks' and never know it, although they may vaguely remember an incident where they felt inexplicably ill and full of foreboding, or had a bout of unusual 'indigestion'. The so-called silent heart attack causes myocardial damage but,

for a time, no noticeable symptoms – and sometimes no lasting problems. Recurrent silent attacks can, however, so damage the heart muscle that heart failure eventually occurs.

People suffering these sorts of attacks, say the cardiologists, may have heart disease which is just as serious and potentially deadly as someone who cannot walk a flight of stairs without chest pain or someone who has been hospitalized for weeks with an unmistakable heart attack. The feeling among experts is that unless these coronary problems are recognized and treated, sufferers are in real danger of a sudden and probably fatal heart attack. Each year, hundreds of thousands of people who had no symptoms die suddenly and are found at postmortem to have had extensive coronary disease.

The effects of silent heart attacks show up on ECG readings and during treadmill exercise stress tests just as clearly as more obvious heart attacks. So why don't we all have routine stress ECGs? Doctors are hesitant to suggest exercise stress tests for every adult. The cost would be high, and many **false-positive results** would lead to unnecessary anxiety and many follow-up tests for a lot of people.

Q **So who should be tested for silent attacks?**

A People who might be at especially high risk:

- previously sedentary men over 35 years old and women over 50 who are about to start a vigorous exercise programme

- men over 35 and women over 50 who have several major risk factors for heart disease – high cholesterol levels, high blood pressure, who smoke, are over-weight, have a high stress level or a family history of heart attack, angina, or sudden death occurring before age 60
- anyone who has suffered a previous heart attack or angina, even though he or she may now be free of symptoms.

Q **How is a heart attack treated medically?**

A That depends on what stage you're talking about. Immediately after the onset of a heart attack, the person needs to be made as comfortable and unconfined as possible: placed in a supine position, with any tight clothing (collars, belts, cuffs, and shoes) loosened. Cardiopulmonary resuscitation is begun immediately if the heart and breathing have stopped. These are measures any of us can and should take to help.

The next step is medical attention. Unfortunately, studies indicate that half of all heart attack victims wait more than two hours before getting help. In heart attack emergencies, injections of really effective painkillers such as morphine sulphate, are given. Intravenous nitroglyc-erin may be started. Depending on whatever other changes occur during this time – blood pressure irregu-larities or arrhythmias, for example – appropriate drugs are given.

The next steps in heart attack treatment are concerned with rest and relief of the anxieties and pressures caused by the heart attack. This doesn't mean flat-on-the-back bed rest in most cases, but probably includes sitting up in bed, resting in a bedside chair or, in due course, some safe and not overtaxing physical activity.

Much of this medical attention may take place in an intensive care unit or a specialized coronary care unit. In so-called uncomplicated heart attack cases, a few days in the ICU or CCU may be followed by as few as three to four days or as many as two weeks of rest, convalescence, observation and medical management in an ordinary ward or separate convalescent area before discharge home. Those with continuing heart and circulatory complications may need a longer stay in hospital; in a few cases, this may include time spent recovering from heart surgery.

Two to three months after an uncomplicated attack, life should be back to normal. Sometimes people condemn themselves to a life of *post*-heart attack invalidism even when they are capable of leading a *pre*-heart attack existence. This is a psychological problem; these people see themselves as in a precarious state, and are afraid to move a muscle for fear of another, potentially death-dealing attack. Unhappily, they may be creating self-fulfilling prophesies. By dwelling on the dark and morbid side, by refraining from activities that promote health, vitality and one's quality of life, they may be hastening the end of their lives. Life is meant to be lived, and if the style of that life – physical activity, diet, psychological outlook – is a healthy one, there is no reason why a first attack should not be the only one, and eventually an event of the distant past.

Q **What is streptokinase? I hear it's a miracle drug for people who have had a heart attack.**

A Streptokinase – as the '-ase' ending indicates – is an enzyme. Streptokinase disintegrates the blood clot blocking the artery to the heart.

Some studies show that, if administered properly and very soon after a heart attack (more effective if given within four to six hours after onset), streptokinase not only can keep heart muscle damage to a minimum, but may very well save your life. Some research supports the conclusion that it is of some value even if given within 18 hours after onset of a heart attack.

That's what some studies show. Others show the opposite – that streptokinase doesn't work miracles in the fight against death, and that a lot of its benefit is caused more by its action as a vasodilator over the long haul than as a blockage-buster at the start.

Q **Are there any other similar drugs around?**

A Yes, but ...

Q **But what?**

A One study – believed to be the largest ever conducted to evaluate the treatment of heart attacks – was the very first to compare all the drugs used to dissolve blood clots when a person is having a heart attack.

Researchers found that all three drugs – streptokinase (Streptase, Kabikinase), anistreplase (Eminase) and alteplase (Actilyse, TPA) were equally effective, but that the oldest and cheapest – streptokinase – was probably as good as the others.

As to effectiveness, about 90 per cent of patients receiving each drug survived, and the study found no very major differences in heart function among those treated with the three drugs. However, a potentially devastating complication of all clot-dissolving drug treatment is bleeding, and this is a risk that has to be taken. The main concern is that the drugs may cause strokes by allowing bleeding into the brain. The consensus view, however, seems to be that thrombolytic therapy, in spite of the risks, is well worth while and can save many lives.

Q   **Why is it important to keep the infarcted area small?**
A   Because tissue death is a natural result of an infarct. What happens is that when the infarcted area becomes **necrotic** – that is, when the cells die from lack of oxygen – or even are severely damaged, scar tissue may or may not have time to form. In an uncomplicated heart attack with a small infarct, the scar tissue firmly seals up the damaged area and, although the muscle is inevitably weakened, this does not greatly impair the heart's normal functions.

With a large infarct, matters are much more serious. Heart failure may occur, or a large bulge – a **ventricular aneurysm** – may appear in the softened and weakened area, causing a life-threatening situation for which the only option may be surgery.

Q **Are there any new treatments – maybe in the developmental or experimental stage – for dissolving clots during heart attacks?**

A In late 1991 doctors stopped a heart attack in progress by threading a laser catheter through the victim's arteries and disintegrating the clot and fatty deposit which had blocked the flow of blood in a coronary artery. This case was the first known instance where such a clot-disrupting technique was used *during* an actual heart attack. Quite a lot of research is going on in the use of catheter-guided lasers to reopen blocked coronary arteries in this way. The method is unlikely to replace clot-dissolving drugs in the near future, but could some day become a routine alternative.

Q **So once the clot is dissolved, then everything's all right again?**

A Not quite. Let's say a clot has been dissolved, leaving the coronary artery open to send oxygenated blood to the gasping heart. That's wonderful – except that quite often blood doesn't get to the capillaries which feed the deeper recesses of the heart muscle, and the muscle doesn't end up functioning properly. In addition, the renewed flow of blood (this is called reperfusion) is not without risk. Reperfusion is known to be associated with the production of large numbers of damaging chemical groups called *free radicals*, which can be very destructive to heart muscle cells. Some early research suggests that it may be possible to protect against the effects of these free radicals with large doses of the antioxidant vitamins C and E.

Furthermore, clots can readily re-form in portions of arteries narrowed by the accumulation of atherosclerotic plaque deposits. Without eliminating those deposits – and there aren't many easy ways to do this – a new clot is ripe for forming at the very spot where the first one was dissolved. Clot-dissolving drugs such as streptokinase work about three-quarters of the time. But it hasn't yet been proven absolutely that dissolving the clot makes any difference to the long-term course of the disease.

Q Can you have more than one heart attack at a time?
A No. You have only one at a time, but the attack may be one in a rapidly occurring series. In fact, the one you feel, the one that hits you hard, may be merely the most recent attack in a string of them. Moreover, symptoms you feel now may be just the tail end of a weeks'-long attack.

Also, a new heart attack may come right on the heels (within a couple of weeks) of a previous one, and the infarcted area may be the same. What usually isn't the same is the outcome – this new heart attack (called an extension of infarction) can lead to grave complications. According to one study, 30 per cent of those people with myocardial infarctions suffer an extension of infarction within the first day or two of the previous attack.

Q Do hearts stop during heart attacks?

A Quite commonly. This, unfortunately is the major risk. Fatal cardiac arrest is the outcome in about half of all cases, usually before the victim can be got to hospital.

Q What are the chances of surviving a heart attack?

A With a minor attack and no or few complications, you have about an 80 to 90 per cent chance of surviving. With complications, the chance of dying leaps to 60 per cent and higher. Unfortunately, many people have these complications. Of all the millions of people who suffer heart attacks each year, statistics show that only about half survive.

Q How can I prevent a heart attack from happening, or prevent a second one if I've suffered one already?

A As we've said before, coronary heart disease is a multi-factorial thing. It's also difficult to say with conviction that if you do this or that, you'll never have a heart attack or never experience another one.

It does seem, however, that nearly every health and medical expert around will agree that lifestyle changes, including controlling the basic risk factors – smoking, drinking, serum cholesterol, stress, poor physical fitness, diabetes, high blood pressure – will go a long way towards making your heart a happier and healthier one.

You will find more details and tips on these factors in Chapter 4.

Q   **Is it safe to have sexual relations after a heart attack?**
A   The answer is a guarded yes. So many people avoid resuming their sex life, fearful that their heart won't take the rigours of intercourse and they'll have another heart attack and die. Not so, in general. Walking up the stairs to the second floor bedroom in the average house elevates the heart rate more than sex does in 70 to 80 per cent of the middle age men who have had uncomplicated heart attacks. Wait a couple of months or so and talk it over with your doctor before returning to this more pleasant form of physical activity. Don't be embarrassed. It's nothing to be ashamed about.

The greatest problem in post-heart attack sex is not physical but psychological – fear of sudden death, psychosomatic impotence and fear and concern transferred from spouse or sexual partner to the heart attack sufferer. It is reported that of all people alive today who have had heart attacks, sexual activity has decreased or stopped altogether in up to 75 per cent. What's worse, about 90 per cent of heart attack sufferers state that their doctors never gave them information about sexual activity, post-attack.

Therapy – group or private – may be required and clearly can be helpful.

Q   **Do heart attacks run in the family?**
A   If you mean 'Is a heart attack a genetic problem?' then indications do point to a family link. There have been a number of studies performed over the years, and they all, to one extent or another, show that if you are a

first-degree relative (for instance, a child) of someone who suffered a heart attack around or before the age of 50, your chance of having a heart attack is significantly increased. One study puts that chance at two to four times greater than in those whose parent or parents (but usually the father) did not have heart attacks. All of this family history seems to apply more to men than women.

What this means is that if your father had a heart attack, your risk is greater, and that if your brother is having heart problems, you should probably have yourself checked. What it does not mean, necessarily, is that you are *certain* to have a heart attack. If you control the controllable risk factors – especially that of high cholesterol levels in the blood, and especially if you begin controlling them at an early age – you may well beat the odds.

Q   **Is it true that heart attacks in women are on the rise? Why?**

A   Unfortunately, it seems to be true. Heart attack is the number-one killer of women in the Western world; all cardiovascular diseases combined claim at least twice as many women's lives as all forms of cancer combined. For a long time, heart attacks among women were rare – so rare, in fact, that little research has yet been performed looking into why women are less susceptible than men. Genes, less testosterone (the male hormone), lifestyle – all could be important factors.

One possible factor in the rise in female heart attacks

may be that as more women enter the previously male-dominated worlds of business and industry, they are also affected by the stress and tension, unnatural work conditions, unhealthy eating habits and lack of exercise their male counterparts take for granted. Much more significant, it seems, is the rise in numbers of women who smoke. For women under the age of 50 who smoke 30 cigarettes or more a day, the chance of having a heart attack is 10 times greater than among women who have never smoked. About 65 per cent of heart attacks are traced back to cigarette smoking, a habit which can be stopped to avoid a disaster that is almost certainly preventable.

Still, far fewer younger women have heart attacks than men, and the incidence of coronary heart disease in women is less than in men. But after the menopause, women's heart disease risk grows. Oestrogen, or rather the lack of it, is the factor at work here. In the largest study to date – published in the *New England Journal of Medicine* in September, 1991 – authorities found that oestrogen replacement after menopause cut the risk of major coronary disease by 44 per cent, and of coronary mortality by 39 per cent. A question left unanswered by this study was how soon after starting oestrogen a woman might see these benefits. On a cautionary note, other experts warn that hormone replacement therapy should not be used indiscriminately among women at high risk of breast or endometrial cancers.

Q **Is the heart attack rate among men rising or falling?**

A Among those who take their health seriously, it is certainly falling. One study of about 100,000 workers over the period 1957 to 1983 showed that the rate of a first heart attack among male employees dropped from 3.19 per 1,000 to 2.29 per 1,000. That's a significant drop, and was mostly attributed to lifestyle changes and elimination of risk factors. In addition, during the early years of the study, men between 45 and 54 years of age had a heart attack rate of 6.47 per 1,000; by the 1980s, the same age group's heart attack rate had plummeted to 2.83 per 1,000.

Even now, some years after the study, researchers and scientists feel that these figures probably reflect what is happening in affluent societies in general.

Q **Did the heart attack rate go down among all categories of male workers?**

A As a matter of fact, and interestingly enough, no. Among salaried – that is, white-collar workers – the first-time heart attack rate dropped 37 per cent. Among hourly-pay – or blue-collar workers – the heart attack rate also dropped, but only by 18 per cent. A probable reason may be that workers with higher educational levels – presumably this refers to the white-collar group – are more likely to effect lifestyle changes to reduce risks, such as stopping smoking, eating better, exercising regularly, or making other changes that may or may not be within the power of blue-collar workers.

A significant postscript to this research was that,

despite the reduction in first-time heart attacks, there was very little increase in the survival rate of those who did have heart attacks. In the early days of the study, 30 per cent of heart attack victims died within a month; today that number is 24 per cent – a very small drop.

All of which says clearly that the route to take is a lifestyle-changing, preventative one.

Q   **I've heard that having a vasectomy increases your chances of having a heart attack. True?**

A   False. Research has shown that vasectomy causes no increase in the risk. There is no obvious reason why it should.

Q   **I've heard that taking aspirin regularly is a way of avoiding heart attacks. Does it work?**

A   The idea behind aspirin being a heart attack preventative comes from the scientific fact that aspirin keeps platelets (small cell fragments) in the blood from clumping together and helping to form clots. No clots, no blocked blood path, no infarct, no problem. There is a problem, though: studies exist supporting both sides of the issue, each promoting a different theory, proposing varying doses, and claiming or disclaiming therapeutic properties for men, women, both or neither. And all the studies hedged a bit in their declarations, and recommended further research to pin down the facts. It's enough to give a person a good reason to reach for an aspirin – to get rid of the headache caused by reading all this stuff.

Aspirin as a protective got a big boost from a 1983 study that looked at how and if aspirin might affect the heart attack death rate among men with unstable angina. The researchers used a buffered aspirin preparation to avoid causing gastrointestinal problems. What they found when they compared an aspirin-taking group with a placebo-taking group was that the aspirin-takers had 51 per cent fewer heart attacks, plus a reduction in mortality among those who did have heart attacks. Aspirin's protective role in women is uncertain, as it was not studied.

Another big boost for the value of aspirin therapy came in 1988. At that time, results of a major national study provided compelling evidence that aspirin could help control the epidemic of heart attacks, according to the American Heart Association. In the light of this, though, indiscriminate use of this widely available drug is still cautioned against, and we should remember that aspirin therapy does nothing to eradicate underlying arterial disease.

Yet another large national study reported in mid-1991 concluded that alternate-day, low-dosage aspirin therapy greatly reduces the risk of a first heart attack among people with chronic stable angina, a group at high risk of cardiovascular death. In the same year, researchers at Oxford underscored the results of more than 200 studies of aspirin. These studies, said the Oxford team, provide conclusive evidence that aspirin can cut the risk of a second heart attack or stroke by 25 per cent.

Clearly, this is an issue you should discuss with your doctor.

Q **Besides smoking, what are the major heart attack risk factors for women?**

A One is what is called 'surgical menopause' – **bilateral oophorectomy** (removal of both ovaries) at the same time that a hysterectomy is performed. Women who undergo surgical menopause have a much higher incidence of heart attacks, and the chance of having a heart attack increases as the age of the woman at the time of the surgery decreases. In other words, a woman undergoing bilateral oophorectomy at a young age – say, 35 – has a far greater chance of having an attack than someone older having the operation. Early *natural* menopause, however, isn't a heart attack risk, unless menopause occurs before the age of 35 – which is quite rare.

Q **Does everybody who has a heart attack go into intensive care or cardiac care units?**

A No. This is unnecessary. Only those whose condition is unstable or who are seriously at risk need intensive care and monitoring. The evidence suggests that there is little or no difference in mortality rates between ICUs and ordinary wards, and that often people do better recovering from a heart attack at home than in an ICU. In fact, one American study indicates that, in some circumstances, you can be better treated at home if:

- you are elderly and without **hypotension** (abnormally low blood pressure)
- you are free from heart failure, or persistent pain
- the heart attack is uncomplicated and you are seen by a doctor some hours after the incident
- your home is far from hospital and you want care at home.

Q **Are there any other 'miracle drugs' for fighting heart attacks?**

A We've discussed one type before: calcium channel blockers, used for angina pectoris. These drugs block calcium from entering the cells in the walls of the arteries, calcium being a primary agent in causing coronary spasm, and coronary spasm being very dangerous indeed. Calcium also causes heart muscle cells to be more 'excitable'.

Another category of drug is the beta blocker, which is used commonly as an antihypertensive medication, as well as for arrhythmias and angina. Beta blockers reduce the heart rate for a given level of exercise and reduce its response to anxiety. By reducing the muscle demand, beta blockers are able to lessen infarct damage. Beta blockers may even bestow an anti-heart attack preventative effect on people taking them for high blood pressure.

The big breakthrough beta blocker was propranolol (Inderal) – which was so effective in one major trial study for helping attack sufferers to survive and avoid second attacks that the study was called off nine months ahead of schedule because it was considered unethical not to give everybody the drug straight away. It reduced mortality by 26 per cent. The researchers weren't sure how propranolol worked. They were just thrilled to have it – and, along with other beta-blockers, it is used a lot today.

Another recent development was a drug called **tissue-type plasminogen activator** – alteplase (Actilyse). This genetically-engineered enzyme was initially thought to work almost twice as well in dissolving clots as streptokinase. But, regrettably, research suggests that it is no more effective, and it is considerably more expensive.

Q **How soon after a heart attack is it safe to start exercising?**

A This is one for your doctor, but, with his or her approval, you may be up and taking some exercise very soon after your heart attack. Exercise, either in hospital or after you get home, or both, is useful in a number of ways:

- It improves confidence and morale.
- It helps to bring to the surface any underlying, continuing heart problems.
- It can aid in forming a better assessment of future action to take regarding your health (including determining if you are a candidate for surgery).
- It prevents muscle deconditioning which occurs during long stays in hospital.
- It can reduce unwanted scar tissue formation in the heart.

What is unclear is whether exercise soon after a myocardial infarction is important in preventing another one.

Q **Do heart attacks happen at certain times more than others? More often during the day? At night?**

A If you have a history of heart disease, the occurrence is spread out evenly, with perhaps a slight rise at night.

Oddly, if you don't have a history of heart disease, beware of Mondays. In a 32-year University of Manitoba study of 4,000 men, the worst, most common day for having a fatal heart attack was Monday. No one knows for sure why this is, though it might have something to do with the stress of returning to work after a weekend of relaxation, or possibly the sudden re-exposure to environmental pollutants.

CORONARY ARTERY DISEASE

Q **What can you tell me about coronary artery disease?**

A We have already covered most of this. The coronary arteries, which bring blood to the heart for its own needs, may become partially clogged with deposits on the artery walls. These deposits are associated with atherosclerosis (the name derives from the words *atheroma*, a fatty mass covered by a fibrous substance and existing as a plaque in an artery wall; and *sclerosis*, a hardening). A blood clot may form on one of these deposits and lead to total occlusion. There are several hypotheses concerning how and why atherosclerosis causes fatty deposits to grow in the artery walls; none has been confirmed.

The acceleration of atherosclerosis – and thus coronary artery disease – may be checked by being careful to control what are called risk factors – actions or conditions found to worsen the condition. The primary risk factors for coronary artery disease, just to remind you once more, are:

- cigarette smoking
- high cholesterol levels
- high blood pressure
- lack of exercise
- diabetes
- family history of the disease
- being male.

The last two you can't do much about, but if you are diabetic you can ensure that the control of your blood sugar is good. The other risk factors are entirely under your control. You will find more detailed information about these risk factors, and how you can eliminate them from your life, in Chapter 4.

We've already looked into the most common manifestations of coronary artery disease – angina pectoris and heart attacks are at the top of the list – and the way they are treated through the use of drugs. Now let's look at a much misunderstood condition: heart failure.

HEART FAILURE

Q   **What is heart failure? Doesn't it mean immediate death?**

A   Not at all. Many people with heart failure live for long periods. In general, heart failure means that your heart is having pump problems and isn't able to keep up an adequate blood circulation and oxygen transmission to the rest of the body. More specifically, it has to do with failure of the heart muscle or defects of the valves, and can affect mainly the right or mainly the left ventricle. When the heart fails, water and sodium are inadequately eliminated from the body, and this can cause severe fluid retention (oedema) and overload.

Q   **How does it happen?**

A   The muscle of the ventricles doesn't have enough strength to contract properly, so that the heart is unable to pump blood out fast enough. What causes the initial ventricular problems usually falls into one of two categories: either there is a mechanical obstruction or blockage of some sort, as with **aortic stenosis** (a narrowing of the valve so that there is obstruction to the flow of blood from the left ventricle to the aorta); or damage to the heart muscle with resulting replacement of muscle tissue by non-contracting fibrous tissue, caused by inadequate coronary artery flow.

Q   **What are the symptoms of heart failure?**
A   Failure of the left side of the heart means that blood
    from the lungs can't be pumped away. The result is
    congestion of blood in the lungs and fluid retention
    there (**pulmonary oedema**). This leads to severe
    breathing problems. As the condition worsens – as the
    left ventricle pumps less and less well or effectively –
    frightening breathlessness, along with coughing, are
    common. At first, physical exertion brings on attacks of
    wheezing and shortness of breath, but later, as the situa-
    tion worsens, these attacks can occur even when the
    person is relaxing or sleeping.

    When the right side of the heart fails, blood stag-
    nates to a varying degree in the lower parts of the body
    and the oedema becomes more generalized. There is
    swelling of the ankles, legs and lower back and an accu-
    mulation of fluid in the abdomen. Liver pain, caused by
    excess fluid retention, is also a symptom of right-sided
    heart failure. Diminished urination may indicate an inad-
    equate pumping of blood to the kidneys.

Q   **What can be done about it?**
A   First of all, your body does all it can to overcome the
    difficulties. Its responses are called 'compensatory mech-
    anisms'. Unfortunately, although these will often work
    for a time, they usually end up causing further trouble.

Q   **What are these 'compensatory mechanisms'?**
A   For one, since the heart's contractions are too weak, the
    body tries to improve the heart's performance by build-

ing up its muscle mass (a situation known as **hypertrophy**). The idea is that more muscle means more power behind each heartbeat. The trouble is, the new muscle creates a need for additional oxygen, just to feed itself. And this at a time when the heart isn't doing a good job of getting oxygen out to body parts that need it desperately.

Also, in trying to maintain the circulation, the heart rate becomes unduly fast and inefficient. This is called tachycardia. The heart rate may also become irregular.

Then, too, there are what are called peripheral mechanisms – attempts by systems not located within the heart to get things back to normal. Among these is the narrowing of arteries and veins. The body brings this about for a simple reason: if the amount of blood being ejected from the heart is low, a narrower pathway will keep the blood pressure up.

Q **So what if I have heart failure? What kind of treatment is available?**

A The normal therapeutic path often starts in hospital, where doctors try to stabilize your deteriorating condition. All possible remedial causes of failure are treated. **Anaemia** can be detected and corrected. Thyroid gland over-activity can be put right. Heart valve disorders can be corrected by surgery. Certain arrhythmias can be eliminated by implanting a pacemaker. But before any of this is done, your general condition can usually be greatly improved by getting rid of excess fluid in the lungs and in the body.

You'll probably be put on a very low-sodium diet, to help reduce the retention of fluid and to keep blood pressure down.

Q **And drugs?**

A Yes, and drugs. Digitalis (often in the forms called digoxin or digitoxin) is the drug most often prescribed for this condition. This drug, made from the dried leaf of the plant *Digitalis purpurea* (purple foxglove), works to strengthen the heartbeat and slow it down, and reduces the size of the enlarged heart so typical of congestive heart failure. Digitalis makes the affected heart a more efficient pump.

In addition, artery-widening drugs (vasodilators) may be used to allow blood to flow more freely from the heart through the body. Common and familiar vasodilators are nitroglycerin, minoxidil (Loniten) and hydralazine (Apresoline).

A most important group of drugs used in heart failure are the diuretics. These are taken to eliminate excess fluids from the body. Diuretic brand names which are widely known include Burinex, Dyazide, Hydrosaluric, Lasix and Moduret. Vasodilators and diuretics are also commonly used to help reduce high blood pressure. Other drugs used to help in heart failure are the selective alpha-blocker vasodilator prazosin (Hypovase) and the ACE inhibitors captopril (Acepril) and enalapril (Innovace). These drugs are covered in more detail below.

You have to really be careful when using any drug,

and these are no exception. This is particularly so with digitalis – especially if you are dosing yourself at home – because its toxic dose is so close to its effective (therapeutic) dose. A little heavy on the digitalis, and you're back in hospital, this time with digitalis poisoning. Among some of the signs of digitalis poisoning are:

- diarrhoea and vomiting
- confusion
- blurred or colour-distorted vision
- depression
- a suddenly decreased heart rate
- dangerous arrhythmias.

Digitalis use may also lead to potassium deficiency – especially if the digitalis is taken by someone who is also taking a thiazide-type diuretic – so it's probably wise to take a potassium supplement, in potassium chloride form, at the same time.

There are other digitalis-drug interactions, and so many ways digitalis use can be risky. A person prescribed digitalis should know why it is being prescribed, should be well informed by a medical or pharmacy professional about the proper doses and uses and about risks, and should be educated to recognize the early signs of digitalis poisoning and how to remedy it.

Q **Are there any new pharmaceutical developments on the horizon?**

A A class of drugs used to treat congestive heart failure

has been found to be capable of preventing the onset of the trouble in the first place. Experts say the findings of this landmark study could lead doctors to prescribe the drug enalapril to hundreds of thousands of patients (although it was also reported that the findings would apply to other drugs in the same class as well). Enalapril, marketed by Merck as Innovace, is one of a relatively new class of drugs known as angiotensin converting enzyme (ACE) inhibitors. These are drugs which interfere with the conversion of an inert natural body hormone called angiotensin I into its highly active form angiotensin II. The latter is a powerful substance which causes the arteries to constrict and the blood pressure to rise. ACE inhibitors prevent this conversion so the blood pressure stays down. They are widely used to treat high blood pressure and advanced heart failure.

Researchers studied more than 4,000 people with mild to moderate congestive heart failure and found that those given the drug were 37 per cent less likely to develop serious heart failure. In addition, there were fewer fatal and non-fatal heart attacks among people taking the drug. While this idea is still rather new, it's worth talking over with your doctor.

CHAPTER THREE

BYPASS AND THE ALTERNATIVES

Q **What happens during a bypass operation?**

A In this procedure, which was developed back in the mid-1960s, a vein is removed (or 'harvested', as doctors like to say) from the person's leg, possibly the thigh, and is used as a detour around the blocked portion of the affected coronary artery branch or branches. It is quite common for three, or even four, coronary artery branches to be bypassed during the same operation. The procedure is simple in principle: one end of the vein is sewn into the aorta and the other is sewn into the coronary artery, 'downstream' from the obstruction, allowing the free flow of blood. Another bypass method is one in which the internal mammary artery, which carries blood to the chest wall and other structures, is linked up with the coronary artery. Many experts consider this method the graft of choice for most patients with extensive coronary disease, although it, too, has some limitations.

For years surgeons have searched for a synthetic

material that could be used, but so far no satisfactory substitutes for human tissue grafts have been found.

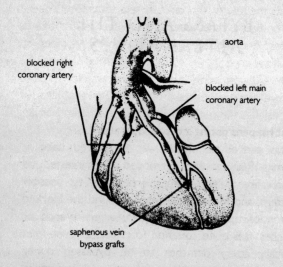

blocked right coronary artery

aorta

blocked left main coronary artery

saphenous vein bypass grafts

Q **Is there any age limit for getting a bypass?**

A It seems not. Study after study indicates that while bypass in its early years had a less than glowing operative mortality rate for older people (around 13 per cent), it is now down to an average of 5 per cent or less. True, while mortality rates for this procedure have fallen steadily since its invention – current literature notes that overall operative mortality of 0 to 3 per cent can be achieved with current techniques – it is best to remember that, as for all surgery, mortality rises with age, with the number and severity of coexistent diseases, and with the presence of any medical problems likely to be adversely affected by anaesthesia. It is also best to bear in mind that this overall mortality rate reflects the results with carefully selected patients operated on by the most experienced surgeons in the best centres. And mortality increases with the number of vessels replaced.

Nevertheless, some surgeons and cardiologists hold that age alone is no reason to deny heart patients in their eighties the potential relief and prolonged lifespan that bypass surgery offers. In one series of nearly 200 people over 80 who had had either angioplasty or bypass surgery, it was found that their survival and complications rates were similar to those of younger people having the same operations.

Most people in various studies who received bypasses claimed that their angina disappeared or much improved. Five-year survival following surgery, even in patients over 65, can be over 95 per cent. However, it is worth noting that, in one of the largest studies conducted, 10-year follow-ups showed no statistically significant difference between survival after medical treatment and survival after surgical treatment. The sole exceptions were in certain subgroups of patients who quite clearly did far better with surgical than with medical treatment.

Recurrence of angina, to a similar or lesser extent, does affect elderly coronary bypass patients, and so does the need in some cases for reoperation due to atherosclerotic growth in the newly grafted blood vessels. Normally atherosclerosis cannot occur in veins; but in these cases, in which veins are used to replace arteries, the disease occurs quite commonly. One advantage of using the internal mammary artery instead of veins is that, oddly enough, the artery seems to be relatively immune from developing atherosclerosis.

Clearly, bypass is not something to be entered into lightly, without lots of information and perhaps a second opinion – no matter your age.

Q **Men and women seem to differ greatly when it comes to heart disease. Are they different when it comes to bypass surgery, too?**

A The evidence points that way. But in this case, the women come out rather worse. According to researchers, being a woman is the third greatest risk factor involved in death from bypass surgery, coming right after older age and having a 90 per cent or worse obstruction of the left main coronary artery.

Far fewer women than men have bypass operations.

Q **What are some of the more serious side-effects of bypass surgery?**

A There have been reports that some people experience conduction problems, some as serious as complete heart block. No one is quite sure why.

At least as serious, and more prevalent, is damage to the brain and memory. Whether it affects long- or short-term memory, this seems to happen frequently enough to worry many medical researchers. After bypass surgery many patients have difficulty concentrating and remembering, and suffer an apparent drop in intelligence. Many find that this problem clears up in a month or two. Others find it does not. In one study, 12 per cent of bypass patients suffered memory loss or other brain malfunctions for short or long periods of time. Preliminary results of an international study show that bypass surgery produces subtle, long-lasting impairment of mental performance in nearly one in five people who undergo the procedure. These findings, however, are still under review.

Q **Why does this happen?**
A Well, it seems to be a problem likely to attend most major heart surgery, not just bypass operations. There are many theories as to the cause. Some doctors think the trouble has to do with the heart-lung machine and with what happens to the blood when it is circulated away from the body, through the machine, then back into the body. Some investigators suggest it has to do with the tubes the blood passes through – they could have bits of contamination or they may generate tiny bubbles that get into the brain – or perhaps it's something called 'protein sludging'. Others think that bits of atherosclerotic plaque break off from the arteries and float to the brain. Whatever it is, it happens, and many doctors either don't know about it or don't tell prospective bypass and open-heart surgery patients about it.

Stroke, during or immediately following the operation,

rose in frequency from about 0.57 per cent to 2.4 per cent over the period 1979 to 1983, due largely to the rising age of patients being operated on. A 1988 study showed a risk of 2.9 per cent for patients who had a prior history of stroke and had general anaesthesia for *any* surgery. Other studies have found similar stroke rates and found that the probability of stroke correlates very highly with the increasing age of those having bypass surgery.

Another mentally related result of bypass surgery is the kind of depression and unfounded fear that causes patients to become invalids, in a manner similar to what we've mentioned about heart attack survivors. Despite the rosy picture painted by many of the strongest supporters of bypass surgery, a large percentage of bypass recipients never go back to work even though their pain is reduced. Further, many become sexually inactive.

Those most severely affected psychologically after the operation tend to be those who were in the worst shape physically before the operation; they thus had a long time to develop a poor self-image and a depressed attitude, which even obvious physical improvement may fail to eliminate. Also, those with good jobs and high status tend to return to work more often than those with low-status jobs. Whether this has to do with white-collar workers who can resume desk work versus blue-collar workers afraid or unable to do lifting and pulling is uncertain, but possible.

Other side-effects or complications include infections

at the chest incision and in the leg at the site of the stripped vein.

Q **Who should undergo bypass surgery?**

A There are some who believe nobody should (we'll discuss them in a moment). In general, however, doctors believe that people with angina so severe that they can barely move without an attack are prime candidates, as are those with serious narrowing of the left main coronary artery, no matter if the symptoms are serious or not, because the person is at risk of sudden death or heart attack. The narrowing can be confirmed by coronary angiography. Some surgeons will go ahead with bypass operations if the person has only mild or moderate angina symptoms and two or three coronary arteries narrowed with atherosclerotic deposits. It is felt by these doctors and researchers that longevity is increased and quality of life is improved by having a bypass under these circumstances. A highly diseased ventricle may, however, rule out a bypass.

Be sure to get a second opinion, and be sure to ask whether alternative procedures, such as balloon angioplasty, would be preferable.

Q **Once you've had a bypass, do the new blood vessels stay clear and free for the rest of your life?**

A Regrettably, no. Even in successful cases, the new vessel or vessels may close, requiring more surgery. The metabolic factors that caused the atherosclerosis in the original arteries to begin with are probably still present –

bypass doesn't cure the disease, it alleviates the symptoms – and this is certainly so if lifestyle changes aren't initiated.

The disturbing post-bypass statistics are that 10 years after the operation about 40 per cent of grafted veins are clogged up again, and 50 per cent of those not shut off are narrowed. One study found blockage to one degree or another in every single grafted vein seen in postmortem examinations of 46 people who had had a bypass operation one to 14 years before. Further, the progression of coronary artery disease is not influenced by surgery, and the incidence of angina even five years after surgery has been reported as being as high as 35 per cent.

This is serious not only because of the recurrence of anginal pain, but because a second bypass operation to undo the failing first is technically more difficult, the chance of death during or soon after the operation greater, and the relief of angina symptoms – seemingly so dramatic after the first operation – less pronounced.

Indeed, there is considerable evidence that the bypass operation itself may cause atherosclerosis to accelerate. While this may be a risk that needs to be taken, it suggests that coronary arteries with minimal disease should not be bypassed. A study from the Departments of Medicine and Preventive Medicine at the University of California at Los Angeles underscored the atherosclerotic danger of bypassing coronary arteries with minimal narrowing (minimal narrowing being defined as less than 50 per cent narrowing of the artery). This study looked at 85 men who had had a graft of some of their coronary arteries, but not all. After three years, the researchers found that the steady progression of atherosclerosis was more than 10 times as common (38 per cent versus 3 per cent) in bypassed arteries as in arteries that were not bypassed.

Q   **Will having a bypass after a heart attack prevent future heart attacks?**

A   No. Many studies show that those who receive a bypass after a heart attack have as great a risk of having another attack as those sufferers who don't have a bypass. Bypass recipients don't live any longer than those who do not have a bypass, either.

The possibility that a preventative bypass will avert a first heart attack has never been established absolutely.

Q   **What are the alternatives to bypass operations?**

A   They fall into four general categories:

1   drug therapy
2   balloon angioplasty and experimental laser angioplasty
3   self-help
4   the controversial chelation therapy.

DRUG THERAPY

Q **Is drug-taking a viable alternative to bypass surgery?**

A One major study says yes. This research looked at 780 people who had either mild angina or a heart attack but no subsequent angina, and compared those who underwent bypass surgery with those who were treated medically. What it found was that there was no significant difference in mortality or in the occurrence of heart attacks between the two groups. The study report suggested that people with mild angina or a recent heart attack with no angina could put off thoughts of bypass until the day, if ever, when their condition had deteriorated to the point where they needed surgery. What mattered was that these people would probably suffer no health penalty for the delay.

While 23.7 per cent of those in the study who took only medicine eventually did have surgery (at a rate of 4.7 per cent a year over five years), the average delay was such that, had they had bypass when it was first recommended, they might already have been having a second bypass, along with its greater mortality risk. This danger was avoided and the operation was performed at the optimum time.

The report admitted, however, that while surgery doesn't add years to patients' lives, it may provide greater angina relief, require less anti-anginal medication, and reduce pain during exercise better than drugs alone. On the other hand, these benefits of surgery – so-called 'quality of life factors' – didn't cause bypass recipients to have more enjoyable leisure-time or to get back to work more quickly than the medication group. It recommended that bypass should be restricted to cases of 70 per cent or greater blockage of the left main coronary artery (that is, only about 1.5 per cent of cases) and to people with debilitating angina which does not respond to medical treatment. Bypass should not be used on people with no or only mild symptoms who have a blockage in only one coronary artery.

Q   Which are the drugs used instead of bypass?
A   These are discussed in Chapter 2: nitroglycerine and other nitrates, calcium channel blockers, and beta blockers.

BALLOON ANGIOPLASTY

Q   How does a balloon help my coronary arteries? What's the procedure?
A   The true medical name for the balloon procedure now being performed many thousands of times a year in place of bypass surgery is **percutaneous transluminal coronary angioplasty** – but let's just call it balloon angioplasty.

In this procedure – developed by Swiss doctor Andreas R. Gruentzig – a plastic catheter tube with a tiny (deflated) balloon at its forward tip is inserted into the groin area and delicately pushed through the femoral artery and up to the openings of the coronary arteries immediately above the heart. It is then turned down one of the main coronary arteries and threaded along until it almost literally bumps into the coronary artery blockage. At that point the balloon is inflated. In effect, it squeezes or mashes the obstruction up against the artery wall, to clear a path for blood to resume travelling along. The balloon is deflated again, it and the catheter are removed and that's it. No chest scar, no stripped leg, no open chest. In some instances, especially after a heart attack, streptokinase is used in combination with balloon angioplasty to clear the arteries even better.

Q   **How long does it take to recover from a balloon angioplasty operation?**

A   Most people who have uncomplicated angioplasties are up and around the very next day, and home the day after that.

Q   **How does the success rate compare with bypass? And how about complications and setbacks?**

A   Figures vary from hospital to hospital, depending on the expertise of those performing the procedure and on how often the procedure is done there. Despite the feeling among some doctors that angioplasty should be limited to cases where only one coronary artery was involved, multiple angioplasty can be performed successfully. In such cases, the most occluded artery is 'ballooned' first. Success in squashing the artery wall deposits was nearly 90 per cent, and more than 92 per cent of patients showed a marked improvement in coronary blood flow.

Fewer than 3 per cent of patients suffered side-effects during the procedure that were serious enough to require emergency surgery. (Sometimes a spontaneous occlusion occurs during balloon angioplasty, and the person needs to be taken for immediate bypass surgery instead.)

The mortality rate for balloon angioplasty is about the same or less than that for bypass – about 1 per cent – although this too differs according to the severity of the disease and other factors. After 15 months, 80 per cent of angioplasty patients report that their angina is completely gone or greatly reduced.

The study also showed that repeat angioplasty for arteries that clog up again is at least as safe as, or probably safer than, repeat bypass. In this study, 37 out of 40 second or third angioplasties were successful.

It should be mentioned that it is too hazardous to do a balloon angioplasty on a left main coronary artery, unless pulmonary or systemic diseases make the person a poor risk for bypass surgery.

Other trials of balloon angioplasty showed that a small, relatively recent obstruction is best for 'squashing' successfully. An old, hard, calcified plaque can splinter, and tiny particles of hardened deposit can float through the bloodstream and do harm by lodging in the brain or lungs. Re-stenosis – when the newly opened vessel becomes narrowed or constricted again – remains a major problem. However, research into strategies to inhibit re-stenosis is currently underway at various centres.

According to some cardiologists, balloon angioplasty is a safe and effective treatment for octogenarians with coronary artery disease. In a study of patients whose mean age was 82.4 years, 81 per cent experienced no further cardiac events – such as death, heart attack, or bypass surgery – in the year following balloon angioplasty, and 78 per cent remained free of such events after three years.

Q   **What about 'preventative angioplasties'?**

A   This is not an option. Like so-called preventative bypass – used to prevent worse conditions that could crop up later on – preventative angioplasties (used in mild cases when obstructions are less than 60 per cent) don't prevent anything. If you have atherosclerosis, all this supposedly preventative procedure does is postpone a worse blockage and set you up to have a second angioplasty or a bypass in the not-too-distant future. And besides, studies show that such preventative angioplasty increases the risk of a post-balloon heart attack.

Q   **Does balloon angioplasty hurt?**

A   Not much, and certainly not as much as bypass. There will be pain at the site of the tiny incision in the groin where the balloon-tipped tube is inserted, and there will be a feeling of discomfort when the balloon is inflated (you'll very likely be awake during this procedure). The insides of arteries are not supplied with nerve endings, so there is no sense of pain involved with the catheter tube snaking up to the obstruction.

Q   **Any other advice about balloon angioplasty?**

A   Yes: see an expert. Not every doctor performing the procedure has long experience with it. If you are going to have balloon angioplasty, try to ensure, if you can, that the person performing it has done at least 100 of them. Check that the operation is taking place in a hospital with a reputation for being a centre of balloon angioplasty activity and with a good reputation for bypass operations, too. Angioplasty is simple, compared to bypass, but it's not easy, and things can and do go wrong: the artery can crack or be accidentally dissected; the heart can go into sudden arrhythmia; or the artery may go into spasm. So it's obviously a good thing to have a doctor and a skilled surgical team who have seen it all. Also, every angioplasty patient has to be willing to be a bypass patient, because if complications occur, that's what you'll suddenly become, no questions asked.

LASER ANGIOPLASTY

Q   **I've been reading in the papers about lasers being used to clear up clogged arteries and get rid of angina. Can you tell me more?**

A   While **laser coronary angioplasty** is full of promise and may someday replace much balloon angioplasty and bypass surgery, it is still experimental. The theory behind laser angioplasty is simple, straightforward and familiar to those who understand balloon angioplasty: a catheter one-eighth of an inch in diameter, containing a fibreglass light guide, is inserted into an artery and pushed forward to the coronary occlusion. At that point, instead of inflating a balloon, the doctor in charge fires an argon laser beam along the light guide at the fatty deposits clogging the blood path. This can break up the blockage. The small resulting fragments are sucked back up the catheter and removed.

Enthusiasts declare that laser angioplasty will do the trick cheaply, quickly (in experimental trials, arteries were totally or partially cleared in under five minutes) and with minimum pain, and people undergoing it without complications can expect to be out of the hospital in a day. In this way, it is favourably compared to balloon angioplasty, and is seen as better than bypass for many arterial conditions.

Q   **Is it safe? Won't the laser just burn up the whole artery?**

A   Again, it's too early to say. In early human clinical tests, the results have been mixed. Most of the cases have ended up in bypass (some out of pure safety concerns for the patient, others because that was what was planned all along), and there have been instances of damage to and even perforation of the artery wall, although in at least one instance it was the catheter tube itself, and not the laser, that caused the injury.

A 1990 report quoted some surgeons, radiologists and cardiologists who use laser angioplasty as saying that the high hopes once held for the technique were not being fulfilled. The main dangers, according to these critics, are the high mishap rates. Any new procedure in its early stages is liable to experience setbacks; results often get better as more are performed. Hopefully, the difficulties will be ironed out. But at present it's too early to say.

SELF-HELP

Q **I've read somewhere about an American magazine editor who refused to have a bypass operation and cured himself, without doctors. Who was it, and how did he do it?**

A You're almost certainly referring to the late writer-editor-lecturer Norman Cousins who, at the age of 65, had a heart attack (he'd had a 'silent attack' some years before). At the suggestion that he undergo bypass surgery, Cousins decided to put that idea on the back burner, and instead see if he couldn't bring himself round by slowing down his work pace, eating better, avoiding stress, and making other lifestyle changes.

Cousins was in a position to trust this self-reliance system: not too many years before he'd had faith in his own healing powers – 'the power of positive thinking' – and in his relationship with his doctor and had beaten the odds (and startled the doctors) by recovering from a serious collagen disease called ankylosing spondylitis. That time, he had pushed fear out of the picture – calling it 'an assassin of recovery' – had buoyed his spirits by watching old comedy programmes and films, had taken megadoses of vitamin C, checked out of hospital and into a hotel, and was lucky enough to have an understanding and helpful doctor. He recovered.

The other time, after the heart attack, he applied many of the same principles, plus walking exercises and other approaches. He made tremendous progress and, in one year, while not back to normal and certainly not completely healed, he was back at work, walking six miles a day, his cholesterol level down, back to his tennis game. He found a way to bypass the bypass, or at least had postponed it for a long time while enjoying a high quality of life.

Now, not everyone can benefit from this course of action; maybe only Norman Cousins could. He had experience and confidence on his side. He also had money and the kind of leisure time away from the job that a relatively monied lifestyle can buy. He was famous, so doctors treated him with respect. They gave him as much information as he desired.

If we all had such privileges, maybe more of us could avoid bypass or balloon angioplasty. Even without these privileges, perhaps we can. For more details about his struggles and victories over disease, we refer you to two of his books: *Anatomy of an Illness as Perceived by the Patient* and *The Healing Heart*.

CHELATION THERAPY

Q   **What exactly is chelation therapy? It is really a non-surgical cure for heart disease?**

A   To 'chelate' means to clamp onto, the way a crab's claws lock around something. In chelation therapy a certain chemical substance – ethylenediamine tetra-acetic acid (EDTA) – is fed intravenously into the body, with the claim that this substance then chelates the calcium deposits that can be found in clogged arteries. Once EDTA binds with the calcium, so the theory goes, it helps to shift the calcium out of the artery walls and eventually entirely out of the body itself through excretion by the kidneys. And thus, according to people (mostly in the US) who employ EDTA chelation therapy as part of their practices, blood is able to flow freely again through the now unobstructed or less-obstructed arteries. Bypass surgery and other invasive procedures can, they claim, be avoided. In the US some 300,000 people are said to have undergone chelation therapy, many to avoid surgery, others as a last resort when surgery was not possible in their cases.

Q   **What does the medical establishment think of chelation therapy?**

A   Not much. Chelation is widely used, and used success-fully, in a number of other completely different condi-tions in which the trouble is caused by an excess of metals such as lead, iron, copper and calcium in the body. But nearly all doctors consider it a potentially dangerous waste of time and effort in coronary artery disease. A little knowledge of the pathology of atherosclerosis will help you to understand why. The plaques of atheroma that cause narrowing of arteries and promote clotting consist largely of fatty material including cholesterol, degenerate muscle cells and fibrous tissue. In advanced cases, the plaques become altered by haemorrhage and ulceration and, at this stage, calcium may be deposited in them. But it is not primarily the calcium that is causing the problem. The notion that the removal of this calcium by chelation would significantly improve the patient's condition is simply not in accordance with the facts. Animal studies have shown that some of the calcium *can* be removed by EDTA, but, according to the *British Medical Journal*, '...there is no acceptable evidence that chelation therapy with EDTA is effective in treating human atherosclerosis'.

The American College of Physicians and the American Heart Association were equally unenthusiastic. The latter stated, in part: 'After reviewing the evidence collected on chelation therapy for atherosclerosis, the American Heart Association concludes that the benefits claimed by this therapy are not scientifically proved [and] recommends that the therapy not be widely applied until it has been rigorously tested in properly controlled clinical trials.'

Another thing that upsets orthodox practitioners are the numerous and varied claims of curative powers attributed to EDTA by its supporters, who say that

EDTA can do everything from saving gangrenous limbs to reducing or eliminating cancers. It is also claimed by some to have an anti-ageing effect. Doctors are also upset that, by choosing chelation, some patients are delaying proven orthodox treatment.

At best, these doctors think that EDTA chelation therapy works as a **placebo**, and that if chelation therapy clinics do anything at all for their patients it is simply that they pay a lot of attention to them, show concern for their ills in a warmer fashion than do many orthodox practitioners, and urge them to follow a healthy exercise and nutrition regimen.

Q **Is chelation hazardous to your health? Is that part of the problem?**

A In addition to the reasons we have already given, doctors base their hesitation and disapproval partly on EDTA's potentially harmful side-effects, which include low blood calcium, bone marrow depression, kidney damage, cardiac arrhythmias, convulsions, hypotension and thrombophlebitis.

Q **If EDTA is so dangerous, why can't it be banned?**

A EDTA does have some medical value – although not in the context of arterial and heart disease. People with lead poisoning or certain disorders of calcium metabolism would be seriously disadvantaged without it.

Q **What do its proponents say?**

A They do not dispute the charges concerning the

possibility of EDTA's serious toxic and lethal effects, but claim that these usually occur only when the treatment has been administered incorrectly (as may also be the case with standard treatment prescribed by orthodox doctors).

Some chelation advocates say that there are good to excellent results in about 75 per cent of patients receiving EDTA, mild improvements in approximately 15 per cent, and no improvement in about 10 per cent.

Q **What evidence backs the chelation proponents' claims?**

A To date, most of the evidence to support EDTA chelation is based on clinical experience rather than on formal clinical trials. There is a distinction: clinical experience refers to the anecdotal evidence and reports of success compiled by individual doctors as they practise medicine. Clinical trials refer to observations collected by means of comparative tests performed under strictly controlled conditions. In modern medicine, clinical experience is valuable and often highly persuasive, but clinical trials always have the final say.

Recent research, while not demonstrating chelation's effectiveness beyond a shadow of a doubt, suggests that it merits further clinical investigation.

Q **What can I do if I want to learn more about chelation?**

A Talk to your doctor about it, but don't be too surprised if you find that he or she has never heard of chelation therapy for atherosclerosis. The official British attitude to this somewhat off-beat subject is perhaps best illustrated by the fact that, in the very detailed, six-monthly indexes to the *British Medical Journal* between January 1985 and July 1995, we were not able to find a single reference to the use of chelating agents for heart or arterial disease.

Q **Is anything new looming on the horizon concerning the treatment of coronary artery disease?**

A Yes, something called coronary atherectomy. Like angioplasty, atherectomy is performed in a cardiac catheterization theatre. A catheter with a small rotating blade inside a protective cutting chamber is inserted into the patient's groin and advanced until the window in this chamber is positioned inside the narrowed coronary artery. A tiny balloon is then inflated, and this presses the plaque into the window where the rotating blade shaves it off 'like a curl of butter'. The debris is pushed into a storage compartment in the catheter tip for safe withdrawal.

Supporters of the procedure refer to the minimal hospital stay – usually overnight – following which the patient can quickly resume normal activities. Unfortunately, the design of the new catheter limits its use to only a proportion of people with coronary artery disease. Best current estimates are that 30 per cent of patients who qualify for angioplasty can have an atherectomy instead. It has to be emphasized, however, that the method is still experimental.

HEART TRANSPLANT

Q **How about a heart transplant? Is it a workable alternative?**

A Yes and no. Heart transplants work. Since the first human heart transplant on 3 December, 1967 – performed by the South African surgeon Christiaan Barnard – thousands have taken place. Initially, the results were not very good and a considerable proportion of patients died. A good percentage of others had to have second and even third hearts implanted to keep them alive. Less than half of those receiving implants lived for five years.

Happily, results have steadily improved and the outlook is now very much better. One should not conceal, however, that there are many problems. You have to be a suitable candidate for a transplant – other major underlying illnesses might invalidate you, as may your age.

Let's say you're selected to receive a new heart. You have to wait until the proper donor heart comes your way. Many people selected for transplantation have hearts so diseased that a wait of a month or so may be too long. Hearts come from donors who have just died or who are being kept on life support machines until the removal surgery can be performed. It may be quite some time before a donor that suits your physical needs – blood group, tissue type compatibility and other factors – may become available.

Then let's presume you are lucky enough to get a new heart. There's the problem of rejection – your body's system fighting off what it perceives as a threatening, alien body. Your immune system views this new heart the way it does bacteria or viruses: something to be surrounded and attacked. Plus there are cells and substances in the donor heart's muscle tissue or blood supply which may interact seriously with your own tissues and blood factors. This is called *graft versus host disease*.

To fight off rejection, drugs are given immediately, and these must be continued permanently. The drug cyclosporin, which interferes with the natural rejection process, has revolutionized transplantation. Steroids are also used. But these drugs do, of course, have disadvantages, as they reduce your resistance to infection and cancer. In spite of all this, the five-year survival rate for people who have had heart transplants is now about 80 per cent, and the 10-year overall survival rate is over 70 per cent.

ARTIFICIAL HEART

Q   **Is the artificial heart a real alternative to other forms of heart treatment?**

A   At the moment, no. Any time soon? No.

The quest to find a workable artificial heart has been going on for decades. Different devices using various materials have come and gone. The last such device in the news was the plastic and metal Jarvik 7 artificial heart. What happened when this was used in operations was just the opposite of what results after a bypass: it prolonged life but not its quality. Certainly the recipients no longer gasped for breath or had heart pains, but the first man – Barney Clark – lived a disorientated, hospital-bound life of suffering for 112 days. And William Schroeder, the second recipient, suffered a series of strokes that caused brain damage. The Jarvik 7 artificial heart is no longer being implanted. One of the major problems is that the device produces showers of small blood clots, and these are carried to the brain where they block small arteries and cause strokes. More advanced artificial hearts which can overcome this problem are in the course of development.

Q **Are there any other artificial devices in development?**
A Yes. Experimental machines called *ventricular assist devices* have been used to help to maintain the circulation of a failing heart. Designed, at least initially, for temporary use to assist a weakened heart, the device is a pump that is externally attached to the heart, although in some cases it may be implanted. The device is powered by an external source – electricity and air – although other designs are testing implantable pumps powered by batteries.

More successful, and for some time now quite widely used, is the *intra-aortic balloon pump*. This device is passed into the main artery of the body and, once in place, is quickly inflated and deflated synchronously with the heartbeat so that it greatly assists circulation. This device is used to keep people alive who have severe heart failure until more definitive treatment, including heart transplantation, can be provided.

CHAPTER FOUR

PREVENTION

Q **Can heart disease be prevented?**

A That is the hope, that is the goal. And in many ways that is the reality. Heredity and gender aren't changeable aspects of human life, and catastrophic events such as coronary artery spasm or a thromboembolism can occur suddenly and swiftly among even those of us who think we are perfectly healthy. But the identification and control of certain factors which increase the risk of heart attack and coronary artery disease may prevent problems in the first place, or avert repeated heart attacks. What we can confidently expect is that the avoidance of the known risk factors may so slow up the development of these dangerous processes that, whatever our previous medical history, we can reduce the chances of future heart trouble. It is never too late to do something about it.

SMOKING

Q **Is it really necessary to go into detail about the hazards of smoking? Doesn't everybody know that it's not good for you?**

A You'd think so, wouldn't you? But surveys have shown that about 40 per cent of people either don't know or refuse to believe that cigarette smoking is a major cause of heart disease. A high proportion – up to 50 per cent – of smokers who have heart attacks resume smoking within a month of their attack. After six months the percentage is substantially higher. These people will often excuse themselves on the grounds that they simply don't believe that smoking contributes to heart disease.

So long as people don't know or won't believe that cigarette smoking is a major heart disease risk factor, and so long as cigarette companies continue to advertise and promote their pernicious wares, we must go on trying to persuade people about the dangers.

Q **How hazardous is smoking?**

A Extremely. After more than 30 years of research into the subject, the medical profession has unequivocal evidence that cigarette smoking is a major cause of coronary heart disease (CHD) in both men and women, and that smoking must be considered the most important of the known modifiable risk factors for coronary heart disease. For smokers, the risk of having a heart attack is more than twice that of non-smokers. In fact, cigarette smoking is the biggest risk factor for sudden cardiac death, and a smoker who has a heart attack is more likely to die from it and more likely to die suddenly (within an hour) than a non-smoker.

As if this were not enough to impress the most hardened and determined of smokers, here are some further points. The death rate from CHD in cigarette smokers is 70 per cent greater than in non-smokers, and the risk of death from smoking increases proportionately with the number of cigarettes you smoke. If you smoke two or more packets a day, your chance of dying from coronary heart disease is twice as high as that for non-smokers. Because many people smoke more heavily than this, smokers, as a whole, have up to a fourfold higher risk of sudden cardiac death compared to non-smokers.

Cigarette smoking alone is dangerous enough, but when combined with other risk factors – elevated serum cholesterol and high blood pressure – the danger is multiplied. Smoking doubles your risk of a first major coronary event when compared to a non-smoker. When high cholesterol is added, the risk is fourfold, and high blood pressure makes the risk eight times as great. Looked at in another way: 23 out of every 1,000 people have heart problems with no major risk factors, but with three risk factors present that figure is 189 per 1,000. And the risk is even greater if you have a family history of heart disease.

It is estimated that approximately 30 per cent of CHD deaths are related to cigarette smoking – *more* deaths than result from any other smoking-related disease, including cancer.

So smoking must be considered the single most important cause of unnecessary and premature death. In the Western world it is responsible for almost one in every six deaths each year. No other single, preventable factor exerts a more powerful negative effect on health than cigarette smoking.

The risk is particularly great in women. In one study of a group of female nurses aged between 30 and 55 it was found that smoking as few as one to four cigarettes a day more than doubled the risk of coronary artery disease.

We do not have the same quality of statistics for developing countries, but we do know that young people in these countries are being targeted by cigarette manufacturers, and that levels of smoking are very high. There is no reason to suppose that the carnage caused by smoking is not worldwide.

Q **Do all these smoking statistics apply to cigars and pipes, too?**

A It seems not. Statistics suggest that cigar and pipe smokers are at no substantially increased risk of coronary heart disease – *unless* they've switched to them from cigarettes and continue the habit of inhaling the smoke. If you don't inhale, there should be no very great excess risk of heart disease. You might get tongue or lip cancer, but the risk of heart disease is thought not to be significantly increased.

Q **Does it matter how long you've been smoking?**

A Certainly. The three smoking-related elements which bear strongly on development of heart disease are the age at which you started smoking, how long you've been smoking, and how thoroughly you inhale the smoke.

Q **Even if I've smoked for a long time, will it help me if I quit now?**

A Of course it will. Your body will positively love you for it. So far as sudden heart attack death is concerned there is an almost immediate risk reduction. So far as the risk of having a heart attack is concerned, this falls off more slowly, but it becomes highly significant a few years after stopping. Here's the key statistic: Ten years after stopping smoking the CHD risk of an ex-smoker approaches that of a person who has never smoked.

This also means that you're never too old to give up, a point bolstered by a study at Yale University which concluded that 'smokers older than age 65 years who have been smoking for several decades can benefit from discontinuing smoking'.

Statistics from the Framingham Heart Study – the biggest ever, longest-running heart study – showed that men who developed angina before the age of 60 experienced a fourfold reduction in attacks when they gave up smoking.

It's also been found that even if you delay stopping until after you have had a heart attack, giving up improves your long-term chances of survival.

Q   **Are filtered cigarettes safer than non-filtered ones?**

A   Most studies say no. Switching from non-filtered to filtered cigarettes didn't affect the disease or the death rate, the Framingham Heart Study showed. It might help to reduce the cancer rate, but not the CHD rate.

Q   **And how about brands of cigarettes with low nicotine and carbon monoxide levels?**

A   Research suggests that changing to these types of cigarettes does not reduce the risks of heart attack. The probable reason for this is that people who try low nicotine cigarettes simply smoke more of them so as to get the same nicotine dose. This is the way addictive drugs work.

    Scientists do not believe that nicotine damages the heart and blood vessels, but there is good reason to believe that nicotine may cause heart attacks by its action in tightening and narrowing arteries. Carbon monoxide, too, interferes with the oxygenation of the blood. Since tars and some of the other 3,000 or so substances in cigarette smoke are known to be very damaging to other parts of the body, it seems reasonable to suppose that they are also damaging to the heart.

Q   **How does cigarette smoke cause heart disease and atherosclerosis?**

A   This remains uncertain. We know that the effect of smoking appears to be a direct one leading to coronary thrombosis and sudden cardiac death, rather than an indirect one by promoting atherosclerosis. Possible mechanisms include:

- the effect of smoking on the tendency for blood platelets to stick together and so promote blood clotting
- the artery-constricting effect of nicotine
- the fact that carbon monoxide combines firmly with the oxygen-carrying **haemoglobin** in the blood and thereby reduces its ability to transport vital oxygen.

Fortunately, these effects operate mainly around the time that smoking is actually occurring and for some weeks afterwards, so, unlike the cumulative effect in lung cancer and other smoking-related diseases, the effect on the risk of coronary artery occlusion passes off relatively quickly once you stop smoking. Clearly, however, these three effects are not the only way in which cigarette smoking causes heart disease, and the other effects may be cumulative and are certainly more long-lasting.

There is obviously a complex interaction between the damaging effects of smoking and the constitution and susceptibility of the individual. This may explain why some people who smoke heavily for a lifetime may live into old age with few problems. These people are, of course, the exception to the rule. So strong is the smoker's desire to rationalize and excuse his or her habit, however, that cases of this kind are constantly being cited as arguments against quitting.

Q   **Well, if I shouldn't smoke, how about a good chew of nicotine gum? Is chewing tobacco or taking snuff bad for the heart?**

A   Very likely. The smallest dose of nicotine increases the heart rate and raises the blood pressure. This effect may not be great enough to be harmful to healthy people, but may be sufficient to endanger people with a heart condition.

Q   **If I don't smoke but everybody around me does, am I at risk of getting heart disease, too?**

A   Passive smoking is linked to cancer and pulmonary infections – and certainly to a lot of annoyance and foul-smelling clothes and hair – but the link between this and coronary disease has not been firmly established. What can be said for certain is that we have no reason to be unconcerned about passive smoking. In the words of a recent *British Medical Journal* report: '...exposure to environmental tobacco smoke cannot be regarded as a safe involuntary habit'. Non-smoking men whose wives smoke cigarettes have nearly twice the mortality rate of those whose wives do not smoke.

Q   **Women and men seem to be different when it comes to getting heart disease. Are women as affected by smoking as men are?**

A   Without a doubt. Women who smoke, whether they are young or middle-aged, are at a considerably increased risk of having a heart attack. Research has shown that the risk of heart attack for women under

50 who smoke is five times greater than for women the same age who don't smoke. It is estimated that 65 per cent of heart attacks among women could be prevented if those women gave up smoking. The danger is greater when other risk factors are involved.

A combination of cigarette smoking and the taking of oral contraceptives is particularly risky: women who do both have a 10-times higher risk of suffering a heart attack than women who do neither.

Q **I'd like to stop smoking but it's difficult and distressing. What can I do?**

A It *is* distressing. But dying of heart disease is even more so. Excuse us for getting morbid and melodramatic about it, but every puff is another nail in your coffin, and the sooner you realize this and do something about it, the better.

First of all, you have to want to stop. You have to make a decision and then you have to take it seriously. Get rid of all cigarettes, lighters, ashtrays – everything connected with the filthy practice. Tell all your friends you have stopped. If anyone offers you a cigarette after they understand you have given up, just walk away from them. What they are doing is just about the most unfriendly act they are capable of and you should make them understand that. Don't waste money or time on group hypnosis to stop smoking. Don't bother about evening classes or other so-called aids to quitting. These are just excuses for putting off the vital decision. All you have to do is to stop.

Smoking is a mild addiction and a very minor pleasure. You are strong enough to act decisively in such an important matter. Oh, and don't go around feeling sorry for yourself. Just do it.

HIGH BLOOD PRESSURE

Q   **How dangerous is high blood pressure? How does it affect the heart? How is it controlled? Are there non-drug therapies?**

A   Good questions, important questions. High blood pressure is such a big topic that it deserves a whole book in its own right (see the book in this Thorsons series, *Blood Pressure: Questions You Have ... Answers You Need* for the whole story).

Suffice to say, however, that high blood pressure can be a killer. Elevated blood pressure indicates that the heart is working harder than normal, putting both the heart and the arteries under great strain. If high blood pressure isn't treated, the heart may have to work progressively harder to pump enough blood and oxygen to the body's organs and tissues to meet their needs. And when the heart is forced to work harder than normal for an extended time, it tends to enlarge. A slightly enlarged heart may function well, but one that is significantly enlarged has a hard time meeting the demands put on it.

Arteries and their smaller branches (arterioles) also suffer the effects of elevated blood pressure. Over time they become scarred, hardened and less elastic. This may occur as people age, but elevated blood pressure speeds this process. In short, high blood pressure accelerates atherosclerosis.

STRESS

Q How does stress cause heart disease?

A You are assuming that it does. You may be surprised to learn that this is not an established medical fact. Indeed, most orthodox medical doctors simply don't believe it, or at least don't believe that there is any convincing evidence that stress causes heart disease.

The real trouble is that nearly all the writing about stress is in the popular medical literature, not in the scientific medical textbooks. And there is so much of this literature that sheer volume has become equated with truth. However, a thing that is not true does not become true just because it is said frequently. We all suffer from stress from time to time, and stress is unpleasant. We can't help feeling that it must be doing us harm.

Stress is a natural and unavoidable feature of humankind. It's what keeps us alert and bright and, in the misty past, kept us one step ahead of the predators who saw early humans as the next meal. It is today's type of seemingly unnatural, work-related stress that is said to do damage. In some studies, so-called Type A personalities – aggressive, ambitious, competitive, workaholic, explosive people, who try to cram 18 hours of work into a 12-hour day – have been identified as prime candidates for heart attacks.

The snag is that, in practice, it has proved very difficult to identify these types with sufficient accuracy and in sufficient numbers to be epidemiologically significant. It's the kind of theory that sounds as if it ought to be right; and experience shows that these are the kinds of theories that people will always believe.

No one questions the damaging effects of single highly-stressful and appalling events on those unfortunate enough to experience them. These people – the victims or spectators of disasters, severe injury or loss, even a heart attack – often get what is called *post-traumatic stress syndrome* and suffer physical effects. That apart, you will seek in vain in any respectable medical textbook for an unequivocal acceptance of the suggestion that stress is a factor in causing heart disease. A stressful event, physical or emotional, that acutely raises blood pressure in someone already prone to heart attack or stroke can, of course, cause sudden death – but that is quite a different matter. Such events do not kill healthy people.

Q **OK. I accept that. But stress is still very unpleasant and it worries me. How can I reduce or control it?**

A You can do everything from changing your lifestyle to changing your job or getting married – all pretty dramatic therapies. Somewhat more reasonable in the short run is behavioural therapy to help you to relax.

Be it biofeedback, meditation or taking a deep breath and counting to 10 backwards – or going out and punching a bag at the local sports club or gym – there are many ways to reduce stress. Look into programmes sponsored by local health groups.

All this is especially important if you've already had a heart attack. As one study recently pointed out, heart attack survivors are '...significantly more anxious and depressed, significantly more obsessional, and significantly more socially phobic and withdrawn than the general population ... Such changes ... may sometimes be amenable to wise counselling.' This was underscored by another study which showed that the rate of second heart attacks among patients who received behavioural therapy fell to 2.8 per cent – half the national rate of 6 per cent. Behaviour modification, the study concluded, could prevent thousands of repeat heart attacks a year, and save numerous lives.

Q **What kind of behaviour modification was that study talking about?**

A Nothing drastic – just sensible. Some basics: no smoking, no big fatty meals, no emotional or physical exhaustion, no caffeine or alcohol to excess. Plus, no aggravation, irritation, anger or impatience, and no daft triggering mechanism like going crazy over sport on TV. If your personality will allow it – take it easy. If it will not, it's time you changed your personality.

EXERCISE

Q **What are the preventative benefits of exercise?**

A The benefits of exercise are widely believed, yet still the subject of some controversy as to effectiveness. Despite a lack of real scientific evidence, an exercise programme, ideally organized by a health professional, appears to provide major advantages. Exercise seems to be able to create a good psychological and emotional atmosphere, releasing tension and stress, lowering your blood pressure and helping you to lose some weight.

Exercising the heart and making it stronger can lead to a lower heart rate. This is always good. Some studies suggest that low heart rate may actually slow down the development of atherosclerosis. Such a strong, slow-beating heart is often referred to as 'athlete's heart'.

Q **But can't exercise be dangerous for the heart, too?**

A Yes. Strenuous exercise beyond your own proper limits can certainly be dangerous. Many enthusiasts believe that so long as you exercise, you only get healthier and healthier. This just isn't true. Sudden cardiac deaths occur in athletes, and postmortem examinations usually reveal that death has been due to atherosclerosis. Hard exercising may also lead to arrhythmias, although many doctors feel that such heartbeat irregularities in otherwise fit people are not serious.

What seems to be really dangerous is the odd combination of smoking and exercising. Obviously, some people think that they can neutralize the negative aspects of smoking with the positive values of exercising, especially out in the fresh air. But, specifically in men under age 35, this destructive duo may trigger heart attacks. And isometric exercises for people with heart disease probably should be ruled out altogether. These static, push-and-pull exercises (including weight-lifting) tend to raise blood pressure and increase the heart's demand for oxygen, which may in turn bring about the blockage of a coronary artery so affected by atherosclerosis that a heart attack is likely sooner or later.

Q **What sort of exercise programme should I involve myself in, especially if I already have a heart condition or have had a heart attack?**

A Experts in the field recommend that you ask yourself what you would like to do, because you have to like the activity if you're going to make it a long-term habit – which it has to be for it to be successful and effective. Don't pick an activity or exercise that is boring and that you're bound to give up in a few weeks. It should be a pleasant experience.

If you think you may grow lax, pick an activity you can do with someone else. That person will keep you in line ... and in shape. Choose something you can do even if it rains or snows, or have a ready, indoor alternative. Your programme has to be a regular one. Also, pick a good time to exercise – one that's easy to set aside every day.

It is extremely important that you should start slowly and build up to higher levels. Concentrate on aerobic or low-resistance exercises such as walking, swimming, running, cycling and racquet sports. Exercises should use both arms and legs. If running is what you want to do, start with brisk walking; then light jogging. Don't overdo – begin with a programme that lasts about half an hour, three times a week.

Don't forget that you must warm up before exercising and cool down afterwards. Avoid exercising in cold weather. It is an additional stress factor, and breathing cold air can cause the coronary arteries and muscles to tighten up, reducing the flow of oxygen to the heart. And don't drink ice cold liquids immediately after exercise. Such a coldness suddenly hitting your system may cause arrhythmia problems. Cool or room-temperature liquids are fine.

ALCOHOL

Q Alcohol is bad for the heart? I thought I read somewhere that it's *good* for the heart. Who's right?

A Both are right. Light to moderate drinking reduces the risk of coronary heart disease. Men who are moderate drinkers have been found to have as much as a 30 per cent reduced chance of having coronary artery disease. What scientists think happens is that alcohol raises the **high density lipoprotein** cholesterol – that portion of the total cholesterol picture that's good for your heart health – in a way that somewhat resembles the after-effects of exercise.

Women as well as men benefit from alcohol's protection. Most British studies have examined the effect of wine, especially red wine. Nearly all of them quote what is called the 'French Paradox' – the fact that although the French, as a nation, enjoy a high-fat diet, they suffer much lower levels of CHD than the British. Some have attributed this to the high intake of wine, and some suggest that there are factors in red wine – possibly antioxidants – which help to reduce the development of atherosclerosis. It is now widely accepted that lipoproteins have to be oxidized before the fatty material can be incorporated into the walls of the arteries. If this is so, antioxidant vitamins (C and E) in adequate doses should help.

That's the good news. The bad news is that alcohol is protective only if taken in moderation. Over-indulgence has a distinctly destructive effect. Alcohol in large quantities can cause what doctors sometimes call the 'holiday heart syndrome': a complex of cardiac disorders often featuring irregularity. Chronic alcohol consumption can cause cardiomyopathy and conduction disorders. A few drinks downed in rapid succession negatively affect the muscle fibres of the all-important left ventricle, and may cause permanent damage in the long run. And more than modest alcohol use is especially bad for you if you have a pre-existing heart condition. Further, excessive alcohol intake raises blood pressure in some people.

So have a drink now and then, if you wish, unless there is a good health reason not to. Have a glass of wine with dinner, or a nightcap. But only that. And don't binge on weekends or holidays, or you may pay dearly for it later on.

DIET AND NUTRITION

Q   **All you ever hear is cholesterol, cholesterol, cholesterol. What's so important about cholesterol anyway?**

A   The fact is that constant high levels of serum cholesterol – that is, the level of cholesterol in the blood – are definitely associated with the formation of atherosclerosis and coronary artery disease. This has been shown in numerous research studies.

A recent examination of data from the Framingham Heart Study has confirmed that high cholesterol levels mean increased risk among people recovering from heart attacks. Compared to subjects who had a cholesterol level under 200 mg per decilitre (within a year after their heart attack), subjects with a cholesterol level over 275 mg per decilitre had a 3.8-times greater risk of a second heart attack. As reported in the American *Annals of Internal Medicine* in late 1991, risk of death from coronary heart disease was found to be 2.6 times greater among the higher-cholesterol subjects. The message from this is loud and clear: if you're recovering from a heart attack, it's critical that you manage your cholesterol level. But there's a good deal more to be said about cholesterol.

Q Let's get back to the basics – what is cholesterol?

A A soft, fat-like substance found in all the body's cells. Cholesterol is used to form cell membranes, certain hormones and other necessary substances. Besides being present in human tissues, cholesterol is also found in the bile and in considerable quantities in the blood-stream. The blood transports it to and from various parts of the body. **Hypercholesterolaemia** is the medical term for high levels of cholesterol in the blood.

The liver provides the body with cholesterol in varying amounts. Additional quantities come directly from foods. Foods from animals – especially egg yolks, meat, fish, poultry and whole milk products – contain it; foods from plants don't. Typically the body makes all the cholesterol it needs, so it's not something people need to consume in any great quantity to maintain their health.

The idea that high blood cholesterol is all that matters is much too simplistic. There is much more to it than that. Some people have a large dietary intake of cholesterol and high blood levels, but suffer no ill effects. The real problem is how cholesterol is involved in forming atherosclerotic plaques. This is still not perfectly clear.

Cholesterol is carried in the blood linked to protein in tiny globules called lipoproteins. If these contain a lot of protein and a little cholesterol they are called **high density lipoproteins** (HDL); if they contain a lot of cholesterol and a little protein they are called **low density lipoproteins** (LDL).

Much of the recent research into cholesterol and

lipids (body fats) has focused not so much on total serum cholesterol levels but rather the proportion of high density lipoprotein (HDL) to the total cholesterol picture. What researchers believe about HDL, and what causes health writers for popular publications to call it the 'good' cholesterol, is that HDL escorts excess cholesterol from the body and helps excrete it, while LDL attracts and hangs on to fatty cholesterol and helps deposit it in arteries and cell walls. The way some medical researchers put it is that the problem is not how much cholesterol there is, but how it circulates and what company it keeps – HDL or LDL.

Thus, a high HDL level means less chance of athero-sclerosis and heart disease, and a low HDL or high LDL reading indicates trouble ahead. Exercise and moderate alcohol consumption have been shown to increase HDL levels. The higher the HDL level and the lower the total serum cholesterol level, presumably the more protected you are. Some studies have indicated even a regression in plaque when total cholesterol and LDL are lowered and HDL increased.

There is a problem, though.

Q **Of course, there's always a problem. What is it this time?**

A It's that scientists still disagree as to how to lower total cholesterol levels, and whether limiting cholesterol in the diet helps to any great degree. They agree that people who already have heart disease ought to be on a low-saturated fat, low-cholesterol diet – why risk the chance? – but that's about all they agree on. It's probably wise and generally healthier to eat a low-fat, low-cholesterol diet, just in case.

Q How high is high cholesterol?

A Conservatively, a reading higher than about 200 milligrams per decilitre of blood will probably raise medical eyebrows and earn you further tests.

Q Is there such a thing as a cholesterol reading that's too low?

A Yes. Cholesterol that drops to noteworthy lows sometimes indicates a disease present in the body: perhaps **pernicious anaemia** or **hyperthyroidism**. Also, there is a significant correlation between low cholesterol and cancer, especially colon cancer, but which is the cause and which the effect is a point of some scientific contention.

Excessively low blood cholesterol has also been linked with depression and even a raised incidence of suicide. Several studies of people taking cholesterol-lowering drugs have shown that they are substantially more prone to depression and suicide than are people not on this regimen.

Q So what is a good cholesterol level?

A Again, doctors disagree. Some are on the lenient side and choose numbers which cause their more cautious colleagues to object. Conservatively and safely, under 200 mg/dl – preferably in the 160 to 180 range – is considered a good level for minimum heart disease risk. Don't aim to get any lower than that.

Q **What can I do in terms of diet to reduce my cholesterol level?**

A Even though the jury's still out on the effectiveness of dietary cholesterol reduction in lowering total serum cholesterol – and the role of diet in heart disease altogether – there are some things that might work. Eat fewer calories, because losing weight helps. It isn't as important as other risk factors, but it shouldn't be ignored. Eat foods rich in fibre. You may not be aware of it, but an enormous amount of cholesterol is excreted by your liver into your intestine in the bile every day. Most of this is immediately reabsorbed into the bloodstream. But soluble fibre is capable of binding this cholesterol into a form that cannot be reabsorbed. Any cholesterol held in this way is passed out with the stools and is lost from the body. This is one reason why fibre is so useful.

Eat more fruits and vegetables, and replace animal fats – saturated fats that are solid at room temperature – with vegetable oils such as corn, safflower, soyabean and sesame, which stay liquid. A vegetarian diet may thus be protective, but fish oils are probably desirable. Get yourself a chart of foods and their dietary cholesterol content, and place a ceiling of 300 mg a day on your intake.

The evidence on the harmfulness of coffee is conflicting. Some studies conclude that it is harmless. Others have linked high cholesterol to men who drink three cups a day or more. Besides, caffeine can elevate heart rate and cause arrhythmias. These are not of benefit to anybody with heart disease.

Q **Are there drugs that lower the cholesterol level?**

A Yes, although – as with nearly everything else associated with the study of and research into cholesterol, athero-sclerosis, and heart disease – results have been mixed. One of the more recent, more successful experiments saw a drug called cholestyramine reduce serum levels, but only under very rigid clinical conditions.

Only if dietary therapy and a weight loss programme have failed over the course of a year or so to reduce an abnormally high blood cholesterol level should drugs be used. They should not be the first treatment turned to. There is one circumstance, however, in which these drugs are mandatory. The condition of *familial hypercho-lesterolaemia* – a genetic disorder featuring high choles-terol levels and a very strong tendency to atherosclero-sis, heart attack and stroke – is much too dangerous to leave untreated. Anyone with an indication of unusu-ally high serum cholesterol levels, or with cholesterol plaques around the eyes (*xanthelasma*) should be checked for this condition.

Q **When they aren't talking about cholesterol, doctors seem to go on about triglycerides. What are triglycerides?**

A Triglycerides are the common form of fat in the body, and having a high serum triglyceride reading is as risky as having a high serum cholesterol level. Triglyceride blood levels normally range from about 50 to 250 mg/dl, depending on a person's age and sex. As people tend to get older (or fatter, or both), their triglyceride and cholesterol levels tend to rise. Women also tend to have higher triglyceride levels than men.

Several clinical studies have shown that an unusually large number of people with coronary heart disease also have high levels of triglycerides in the blood. This is called **hypertriglyceridaemia**. However, some people with this problem seem remarkably free from athero-sclerosis. Thus, elevated triglycerides, which are often measured along with HDL and LDL, may not directly cause atherosclerosis, although they may accompany other abnormalities which speed its development.

Q **Do you think antioxidant vitamins are relevant in all this?**

A Yes. The medical literature on the subject is now exten-sive, and much of it seems to be concerned with the now widely accepted view that cholesterol gets into the artery linings when the low density lipoproteins are oxidized by the action of free radicals. If this is true, we may be getting to the root of the problem of athero-sclerosis.

There is a good deal of indirect support for this suggestion. In May 1993, the *New England Journal of Medicine* published reports on two major series of studies, on 87,245 women and 39,910 men respectively. These were followed up for eight years, and the outcome in those with a high vitamin E intake was compared with those with a low E intake. The conclusion was that a high vitamin E intake substantially reduces the risk of coronary heart disease in both women and men.

Q   **So you think I should be taking vitamin E?**
A   Other evidence suggests that both vitamin C and vitamin E are required to produce the fullest protection against CHD and many other free radical-produced disorders.

Q   **OK. So how much should I be taking?**
A   This is not yet completely clear, but it seems likely that 1,000 mg (1 g) of vitamin C and 300–400 mg (or IU) of vitamin E should be enough for adults. The dose of C can safely be increased if necessary. Note that high doses of vitamin E can be dangerous in babies and infants.

Q   **What about high doses of vitamins A and D?**
A   Don't even consider it. These are not antioxidants, and high doses can be dangerous to anyone.

Q   **What is this Pritikin Diet I've heard about? Isn't it supposed to improve the health of people with heart disease?**
A   That's what the Pritikin plan claims, and its proponents have studies to back it up. The programme was developed when the late Nathan Pritikin did some research

and found that, despite the enormous stresses and fear experienced by many European people during the Second World War, the incidence of heart disease and heart attacks was very low. Why? Pritikin and others contended that it was the diet: low in dairy fats – milk, cheese, butter and eggs being difficult to find during the war (as was meat) – and high in fibre and complex carbohydrates. Starting in 1976, Pritikin applied his theories to people who needed help after heart attacks or who wanted to avoid bypass surgery. Many of them who could barely crawl when they arrived at Pritikin's Longevity Centers walked out with the glow of what appeared to be health.

The Pritikin diet is a very strict one, limiting daily cholesterol intake to as little as 25 mg. It also prohibits fatty meats (some fish and chicken are allowed), sugar (as well as honey and treacle), salt, eggs, oils and nuts, among other common staple foodstuffs. Fruits and vegetables and whole grains rule the dietary roost. Cholesterol level reductions of 25 per cent are claimed by Pritikin people.

Many doctors believe the Pritikin plan is a good one, except for one drawback: it is so inflexible and sometimes so bland and unattractive that people have great difficulty in keeping it up and tend to 'fall off the wagon' in search of more tasty food. Complete and long-term compliance is all-important in a heart regimen, and if the programme itself encourages cheating or non-compliance, it can't be considered *the* answer.

Still, even a modified Pritikin diet would undoubtedly

HEART DISEASE

do a lot of good for a lot of people, and it is easy to find such food in supermarkets. One word of warning: If your diet is already low in cholesterol, don't try to cut down too far on this vital ingredient. Remember the risks of excessively low cholesterol levels. Moderation in everything.

Q **I've heard that eating fish is good for the heart. True?**
A True. It's been known for a long time now – scientific publications have been running studies for years – but ever since the prestigious *New England Journal of Medicine* gave it its seal of approval, it's become official: eating fish even once or twice a week may significantly reduce the risk of heart attack.

It's believed to be the fish oils – rich in eicosapentaenoic acid, or omega-3 fatty acid – that do the job, found in saltwater fish such as salmon, tuna, flounder and cod. These oils appear to reduce triglyceride levels and retard blood platelet aggregation, which, in turn, may prevent blood clots from forming in atherosclerosis-narrowed coronary arteries, and causing heart attacks.

But fish oil is no miracle drug. Don't expect to be able to eat poorly and smoke, then cancel it out with a tuna casserole. Eating fish has to be just one element of a good, overall health programme.

Q **Is lecithin a heart disease preventative?**
A The dietary supplement lecithin does no good for the heart, and in some instances may do some harm.

Q **What about vitamins and minerals other than the antioxidant ones? Any of them good to take for heart disease?**

A Yes. But this statement has to be qualified. Vitamin and mineral deficiency is very rare even in people whose diet is relatively poor. So don't imagine you are likely to do much good by taking additional supplements when you are already getting more than your body needs. With this in mind, here's an overview of the most important points about vitamins and minerals:

MAGNESIUM

This mineral has recently been shown to have some medical applications even in people who are not deficient. In clinical studies, magnesium administered during acute myocardial infarction seemed to reduce the size of the infarct and to reduce ventricular abnormalities. So it is now fairly routinely used by doctors, often given by injection and always in carefully measured doses.

Magnesium deficiency has been linked to sudden death in patients with ischaemic heart diseases, the deficiency causing coronary artery spasm. It's also been implicated in ventricular tachycardia (a heartbeat irregularity) and in chronic heart failure.

A rare lack of magnesium in the diet and impaired absorption of it, as well as depletion of it due to digitalis toxicity and the use of some diuretics, can all be factors in dangerous magnesium deficiency. People who drink 'soft' water – stripped of its natural minerals, including magnesium – may possibly be more at risk of heart disease than those who drink 'hard' water. Foods high in magnesium include tofu, soy flour, black-eyed peas, wheat germ, nuts (cashews, almonds, brazil nuts, and pecans), peanuts, and kidney and lima beans.

POTASSIUM

Same story here, and it works in concert with magnesium in a balance with calcium and sodium. It is very unlikely that anyone would be deficient in potassium for dietary reasons, but a low blood potassium level leads to arrhythmias. The presence of potassium in healthy amounts is necessary for certain anti-arrhythmia drugs to work properly. There is often a low blood potassium in people who have heart attacks. Potassium deficiency can be caused by the taking of diuretics, because these usually promote greatly increased urinary excretion of this mineral.

Foods high in potassium include brussels sprouts, cauliflower, avocado, potatoes, tomatoes, bananas, cantaloupe, peaches, oranges, flounder, salmon and chicken.

NIACIN

Once known by the nondescript name of vitamin B_3, niacin is found in a wide variety of foods such as meat (especially liver), chicken, fish (especially tuna and salmon), whole grains, wheat germ, dairy products, eggs, nuts, dried beans and peas. It is usually sold as nicotinic acid or, even more commonly, nicotinamide. Niacin's ability to reduce cholesterol levels in the blood has long been recognized, but since it is a vitamin and cannot be patented, no pharmaceutical company has bothered to test and promote it in the fight against heart disease. However, in 1990 researchers from the University of Pennsylvania reported that niacin was the least costly medication available for reducing cholesterol levels – according to their calculations, it can achieve a 1 per cent reduction for one-third to one-half the cost of other cholesterol-lowering drugs.

Very important to note is the fact that niacin is not without side-effects, many of them potentially serious: they range from flushing, rashes, itching, hives, nausea, diarrhoea and abdominal discomfort to liver malfunction, jaundice, elevated uric acid levels and gout, abnormally high blood sugar levels, peptic ulcers and the aforementioned abnormal heart rhythms. The soundest advice for anyone is not to self-administer niacin in any form or switch the type already being used without consulting a doctor. Further, many experts recommend that people using megadoses of any kind of niacin get liver function tests every few months, as well as periodic checks of blood sugar and uric acid levels.

SELENIUM AND ZINC

These trace minerals are also mentioned frequently as substances that should be found in adequate amounts in the diet (or taken in supplements) to aid in heart health. Deficiency in these metals is, however, almost unknown except in people who are being fed exclusively by the intravenous route. Nowadays, even such diets should contain traces of these minerals.

As mentioned above, *antioxidant vitamins* may turn out to be the most important dietary factors of all when it comes to heart health. (For more information about a healthy diet, see *Vitamins and Minerals: Questions You Have ... Answers You Need* in this Thorsons series.)

CHAPTER FIVE

OTHER QUESTIONS ABOUT THE HEART AND ITS DISEASES

Q I'm taking lithium for depression. Is it harmful to the heart?

A This is not a major problem for people with healthy hearts. But overdosage with lithium can cause certain heartbeat irregularities and conduction problems, and people with heart disease should use lithium salts with caution, if at all. Presumably, if there is any question of your having a heart disorder your doctor will be aware of it. It would be a good idea to discuss this with your doctor.

Q Is heart disease a geographical problem?

A To some extent it is. The incidence of death from heart disease is higher in some places than in others. Scotland, for instance, has a substantially higher rate than the south of England. The explanation for this is not entirely clear. Some epidemiologists have suggested that there is a link between soft water and a high prevalence of heart disease (see Chapter 4). Hard water seems to be relatively protective. Probably more important are general differences in affluence, lifestyle, environmental pollution, even weather.

Q   **Is it OK for somebody with heart disease to travel?**
A   Usually it's just fine, if you're cautious and prepared for untoward possibilities. There are a few points you should bear in mind. Don't travel by air if you have heart failure or have had a heart attack in the previous month. Remember that aircraft are pressurized at a level somewhat below normal and you may run short of oxygen. If you are planning to travel by air, ask your doctor whether you will need supplementary oxygen. If so, you must contact the airline and tell them, so that arrangements can be made. Their medical department will almost certainly want to know more about your condition, and you may have to attend a special examination.

If you are taking a long flight or coach ride, remember the risk of deep leg vein thrombosis from sustained pressure on your thighs. Don't sit in the same position for long periods. Get up and move around frequently, if only to take a walk up and down the aisle.

Do remember that the drugs you need must be readily available to you on a long journey – don't pack them away in baggage you've checked in before the flight. Keep them in your hand luggage, especially if travelling by air. And, talking of baggage, do use porters when you can. In your holiday mood, don't lose sight of your physical limitations and start hoisting 50-pound suitcases around.

When travelling by sea, don't be tempted to drink

too much. Sea voyages may be health-giving, but not if you give way to overindulgence.

Q **Is there any ethnic group more prone to heart disease than others?**

A Not many studies look into this subject, but many of those that do show that Jewish males are at greater risk than many other ethnic types. And black people have an almost one-third greater chance of having high blood pressure compared with whites.

Q **Are there work-related hazards that cause or worsen heart disease?**

A Heart disease is certainly a major feature of industrialized societies, but there is comparatively little evidence of a specific relationship between particular occupations and heart disease. Everyone knows that cigarette smoking, physical inactivity and obesity are risk factors, but these are not necessarily related to any particular job. Some occupations, however, seem to encourage them. Work involving physical activity is protective against coronary heart disease. Unfortunately, many manual workers also expose themselves to avoidable risk factors, as we have already explained.

Exposure to carbon monoxide cuts down the oxygen-carrying power of the blood. Exposure to carbon disulphide and carbon tetrachloride appears to promote high blood pressure and raised blood cholesterol. Workers exposed to nitrates may suffer angina and heart attacks after a short period of absence from work. This is thought to be due to a kind of rebound spasm of the coronary arteries after they have been widened by the nitrates. Halogenated hydrocarbons and fluorocarbons may cause arrhythmias, and these may be fatal. Cobalt can cause cardiomyopathy. More studies need to be done in this area.

Q **Is it dangerous to have an operation which has nothing to do with the heart if you have heart disease?**

A Research suggests that, in people who have had a previous heart attack, general surgery and anaesthesia will cause a new heart attack in about 6 per cent of cases. If the heart attack happened less than three months before surgery, the chance for reinfarction is 30 per cent; if the time elapsed is four to six months, the risk drops to 15 per cent. Among those who have these surgery-related heart attacks, 50 to 70 per cent die within a week.

In one study of 99 people there were no cardiac deaths from non-cardiac surgery among those who'd had a bypass operation. In addition, people who have had valve replacements seem to be in little danger.

Q **Has heart disease always been the number-one killer in the West?**

A No. Its pre-eminence as Public Health Enemy Number One is comparatively recent, coming as a result of the medical control of other illnesses which were once more common. At the turn of the century, heart disease was fourth among killer conditions. Pneumonia and

influenza (that's one category), tuberculosis, and diarrhoea and other intestinal ailments were ahead of it.
Improvement in public health and sanitation, and the
advent of the antibiotics changed all that, and it was not
long before heart disease was at the top of the list.

Heart disease is now, happily, in decline, thanks
largely to greater public awareness of the importance of
a healthier lifestyle.

Q   **When we think of heart disease, more often than not
we think of adults. Do children present special problems when it comes to heart disease?**

A   Earlier in this book we mentioned congenital heart
disorders. These are in a class of their own and require
special medical expertise. It is important, however, to
realize that the origins of heart disease are to be found
in childhood. In our pampered society these origins can
date from infancy. Pathological studies of children's
arteries often show fatty streaks, thought to be the earli-
est stages of atherosclerosis. The moral is clear: nipping
heart disease risk factors in the bud can give your child a
chance of a long and heart disease-free life. Here are
some of the most important points taken from many
studies. They are certainly worth noting:

- Dietary, smoking and exercise habits are established
  early in life. Parents and schools need to be
  educated about heart disease so that they can
  influence young children and encourage heart
  health through example and effective programmes.

- Some doctors and researchers believe tests for serum cholesterol levels should begin early in life, at least by school age, and especially among those male children with a family history of heart problems. In fact, high cholesterol and triglyceride levels in children can indicate that their parents, too, have heart disease they may not know about.

- Some doctors believe that early intervention is more successful than waiting until the child becomes an adolescent or adult. This may make it possible to keep the arteries clean in later life. Such intervention should involve a check for diabetes and should keep track of those children who are obese, physically inactive and/or have already developed high blood pressure.

- Early smoking and oral contraceptive use among children and adolescents under age 17 significantly increase cholesterol and triglyceride levels, and create a heart disease risk at a young age. These should be strongly discouraged.

- A hypertensive father can pass on high blood pressure to his children merely through the behaviour he demonstrates when coping with anger and stress. In tests, the inability of hypertensive fathers to handle situations in the presence of their children raised the children's blood pressure.

- Probably most important of all is the question of diet. When monkeys were fed a typical affluent Western world diet – high in saturated fats, salt and sugar and full of snacks – the poor animals developed high blood pressure. Said one researcher, 'Feeding monkeys the diet children eat is a good model for producing atherosclerosis.'

Q **Does pregnancy present a danger to women with heart disease?**

A It certainly can, especially in women with valvular disorders and congenital heart defects. Late in pregnancy, the increased strain on the heart and lungs can send these young women into heart failure. So if you have a heart problem you should make quite certain that you get lots of information both from the person who will deliver your baby and from a cardiologist.

Remember that antibiotics given during labour and delivery can prevent endocarditis and other bacteria-caused damage in women with valvular disorders.

If you are worried that your child will inherit your congenital defect, discuss your fears with your doctor. Remember that a great many congenital heart defects are *not* hereditary. Ask your doctor about yours.

USEFUL ADDRESSES

British Heart Foundation
14 Fitzhardinge Street
London W1H 4DH
0171–935 0185

British Heart Foundation Heart Research
Langthorne Hospital
Langthorne Road
London E11 4HJ
0181–539 8828

Coronary Artery Disease Association
Tavistock House
Tavistock Square
London WC1H 9HP
0171–387 9779

National Heart and Lung Institute
Dovehouse Street
London SW3 6HP
0171–352 8121

The Coronary Prevention Group
Plantation House
Fenchurch Street
London EC3M 3DX
0171–626 4844

The Stroke Association
CHSA House
123–127 Whitecross Street
London EC1Y 8JJ
0171–490 7999

Health Information Services
Freephone 0800 66 55 44

Health Education Authority
Hamilton House
Mabledon Place
London WC1A 9YT
0171–383 3833

Women's Health
52 Featherstone Street
London EC1Y 8RT
0171–251 6580

GLOSSARY

ACUTE NONSPECIFIC PERICARDITIS

A condition in which the **pericarditis** is not secondary to another disease, but in which the **pericardium** is attacked directly itself by a virus

ACUTE PERICARDITIS

See **Pericarditis**

ANAEMIA

A condition in which the blood is deficient in red blood cells or in **haemoglobin**

ANGINA PECTORIS

The medical term for a severe, suffocating chest pain caused by an insufficient amount of blood being supplied to the heart muscle

ANGIOGRAPHY

An imaging procedure that enables blood vessels to be seen on film after the vessels have been filled with a contrast medium – a substance opaque to X-rays. It is used to detect diseases which alter the appearance of the blood vessel channel

ANNULOPLASTY

A kind of plastic surgery in which heart valve tissue is reconstructed

AORTA

The body's primary **artery**, which receives blood from the heart's left **ventricle** and distributes it to the body

AORTIC STENOSIS

An obstruction to the flow of blood from the left **ventricle** to the **aorta**

AORTIC VALVE

The heart valve between the left **ventricle** and the **aorta**. It has three flaps, or cusps

ARRHYTHMIA (OR DYSRHYTHMIA)

Any abnormal rhythm of the heart

ARTERIOLE

A small branch of an **artery** that links the artery to a **capillary**

ARTERY

A blood vessel that carries blood away from the heart

ATHEROMA

A fatty mass, covered by fibrous substance and existing as a **plaque** in an artery wall

ATHEROSCLEROSIS

The most prevalent form of arterial disease, in which the inner layers of artery walls become thick and irregular due to deposits of fat, cholesterol and other substances. As the interior walls of arteries become lined with layers of these deposits, the arteries become narrowed and the flow of blood through them is reduced. Coronary artery atherosclerosis is the cause of the great majority of cases of angina and heart attacks

ATRIAL FIBRILLATION

A type of irregular heartbeat in which the upper chambers of the heart beat irregularly and very rapidly

ATRIAL FLUTTER

A type of irregular heartbeat in which the upper chambers of the heart beat very rapidly and weakly

ATRIAL PAROXYSMAL TACHYCARDIA

A condition in which the heartbeat suddenly becomes abnormally fast – with beats of up to 220 a minute – then just as suddenly returns to normal

ATRIOVENTRICULAR (AV) NODE

A small mass of specialized conducting tissue at the bottom of the right **atrium,** through which the electrical impulse stimulating the heart to contract must pass to reach the **ventricles**

ATRIUM

Either one of two upper chambers of the heart in which blood collects before being passed to the **ventricles;** also called auricle

BALLOON ANGIOPLASTY

A procedure for treating narrowing or blockage of a blood vessel or heart valve. A catheter with a deflated balloon on its tip is passed into the narrowed artery segment, the balloon inflated, and the narrowed segment widened

BETA BLOCKER

A drug principally used to treat heart disorders such as high blood pressure (**hypertension**), **angina pectoris**, and cardiac **arrhythmia**

BILATERAL OOPHORECTOMY

Removal of both ovaries

BRADYCARDIA

An abnormally slow heartbeat

CALCIUM CHANNEL BLOCKER

A drug used to treat **angina pectoris**, **hypertension** and certain types of cardiac **arrhythmias**

CAPILLARY

Any of the minute vessels that carry blood between the smallest arteries and the smallest veins

CARDIAC CATHETERIZATION

The process wherein a thin, flexible tube is inserted into a blood vessel (usually in the groin or arm area) and is then pushed along the vessel and on into the heart, for the purpose of examination

CARDIAC TAMPONADE

Compression of the heart

CARDIOMYOPATHY

A serious disease involving an abnormality and decreased function in heart muscle

CARDIOPULMONARY RESUSCITATION (CPR)

A technique combining chest compression and mouth-to-mouth breathing, used during cardiac arrest to keep oxygenated blood flowing to the heart muscle and brain until advanced life support can be started

COMMISSUROTOMY

A procedure in which thin heart valve leaves – stuck together because of scar tissue formed after a bout of rheumatic fever-induced **endocarditis** – are separated

COMPUTERIZED TOMOGRAPHY (CT) SCANNING

A computer-enhanced series of cross-sectional X-ray images of a selected part of the body. This test can detect many conditions which cannot be seen in ordinary X-rays

CONGENITAL

Denotes conditions existing at birth

CONGESTIVE HEART FAILURE

A condition in which the heart, as a result of disease, is no longer capable of maintaining an adequate circulation of blood for the body's needs. The result is often breathlessness and accumulation of fluid in the lungs and dependent parts of the body (oedema)

CONSTRICTIVE PERICARDITIS

A condition in which the **pericardium** becomes scarred, thickened and hard, often with calcium deposits. The heart is no longer free to move properly and its mechanical function is interfered with

CORONARY ARTERIES

Two arteries arising from the **aorta** which arch down over the top of the heart, branch out, and provide blood to the heart muscle

DEFIBRILLATION

Electric shocks delivered to the heart so as to terminate an otherwise fatal fluttering and non-pumping of the **ventricles**, and to allow normal rhythm to resume

DEFIBRILLATOR

An electronic device – basically two metal paddles connected to a chargeable electric capacitor (a source of high-voltage electricity) – which helps re-establish normal contraction rhythms in a heart that is fluttering but is no longer pumping blood

DIASTOLE

The lowest blood pressure measured in the arteries. It occurs when the heart is between contractions

DIGITALIS (ALSO DIGOXIN, DIGITOXIN)

A drug that slows and strengthens the contraction of the heart muscle, thereby improving its performance and promoting the elimination of fluid from body tissues

DIURETIC

A drug that promotes urination, thus speeding the elimination of retained water from the tissues of the body. This is an effective and much-prescribed method of getting rid of excess body fluid (oedema). It may also help in blood pressure control

ECHOCARDIOGRAPHY

A diagnostic technique in which pulses of sound are transmitted into the body and the echoes returning from the surfaces of the heart and other structures are electronically processed and represented as images on a cathode-ray tube or other display

ELECTROCARDIOGRAM (ECG)

A graphic record of electrical impulses produced by the heart, used by doctors to help in the diagnosis of a wide range of heart disorders

ENDOCARDITIS

An inflammation of the internal lining of the heart, particularly the valves, because of an infection

ENDOCARDIUM

The internal lining of the heart

FALSE-POSITIVE RESULT

One in which a test gives a positive, or abnormal result when no disease is actually present

FLUOROSCOPY

A specialized X-ray procedure allowing the observation of moving objects such as a catheter in a blood vessel. Without fluoroscopy, a doctor would not be able to place the tip of a catheter where it is needed

HAEMOGLOBIN

The oxygen-carrying pigment found in red blood cells

HEART BLOCK

A disorder of conduction of the impulse for the heartbeat. There is severe slowing of the ventricular contraction rate which may lead to dizziness, fainting, heart attack or stroke

HIGH BLOOD PRESSURE

See **Hypertension**

HIGH DENSITY LIPOPROTEIN (HDL)

A carrier of cholesterol believed to transport cholesterol away from the tissues and to the liver, where it can be excreted

HYPERCHOLESTEROLAEMIA

A high level of cholesterol in the blood

HYPERTENSION

A persistent increase in blood pressure above its normal range. Hypertension is damaging to arteries and is one of the causes of **atherosclerosis**

HYPERTHYROIDISM

A condition in which the thyroid gland functions excessively. General hyperactivity and a fast heart rate are common physical signs of hyperthyroidism. This can add to the load on the heart

HYPERTRIGLYCERIDAEMIA

A high level of fats (**triglycerides**) in the blood

HYPERTROPHY

Enlargement of an organ or tissue resulting from an increase in the size of its component cells. Hypertrophy of the heart is a natural result of an increased work load on the heart

HYPOTENSION

Low blood pressure. Except in extreme cases such as surgical shock or toxic shock this is not considered by most British doctors to be a formal disease, nor to cause bodily disorder

HYPOTHERMIA

A fall in body temperature to below 35°C (95°F)

HYPOTHYROIDISM

Deficient activity of the thyroid gland resulting in under-production of thyroid hormones and a general slowing of all bodily activities

HYPOXIA

An inadequate amount of oxygen to the tissues

INFARCTION

Death of an area of tissue caused by lack of blood supply

INFERIOR VENA CAVA

One of two very large veins into which all the circulating deoxygenated blood drains. This vein starts in the lower abdomen and travels some 10 inches upwards before connecting to the right **atrium**. It collects blood from all parts of the body below the chest

ISCHAEMIA

Decreased blood flow to an organ, usually due to obstruction of an **artery**

LASER CORONARY ANGIOPLASTY

A procedure for treating a narrowing or blockage (**occlusion**) of a blood vessel. A fine catheter containing a fibre optic light guide is inserted into the vessel and pushed forwards to the coronary occlusion. At that point a laser connected to the outer end of the light guide is fired. Laser energy disrupts the fatty deposits clogging the blood path and clears the blockage

LEFT ATRIUM

See **Atrium**

LEFT VENTRICLE

See **Ventricle**

LOW BLOOD PRESSURE

See **Hypotension**

LOW DENSITY LIPOPROTEIN (LDL)

The main carrier of harmful cholesterol in the blood

MAGNETIC RESONANCE IMAGING (MRI)

A diagnostic technique that provides high-quality cross-sectional images of organs and structures within the body without X-radiation. MRI produces especially detailed images of the heart, major blood vessels and blood flow

MEDIASTINUM

The central compartment of the chest, lying between the lungs and containing the heart, windpipe, oesopha-gus, the major blood vessels entering and leaving the heart, lymph nodes and lymphatic vessels, thymus gland and various nerves

MITRAL VALVE

The heart valve between the left **atrium** and left **ventricle**. It has two flaps, or cusps

MYOCARDIAL INFARCTION (MI)

The damaging or death of an area of the heart muscle resulting from a reduced blood supply to that area; the pathological basis of a heart attack

MYOCARDIUM

The muscular wall of the heart. It contracts to pump blood out of the heart and then relaxes as the heart fills with returning blood

NECROTIC

Dead; pertaining to, or characterized by, death of tissue

OCCLUSION

Blockage of any passage, canal, vessel or opening in the body

PARACENTESIS

Drainage of excess of fluid (effusion) from within a body cavity or organ, such as the **pericardium**. Drainage of excess pericardial fluid is sometimes called a pericardial tap

PERCUTANEOUS TRANSLUMINAL CORONARY ANGIOPLASTY

See **Balloon angioplasty**

PERICARDIAL EFFUSION

An abnormal collection of fluid between the heart and the pericardial sac that encloses it. The fluid is usually the result of excessive secretion by the inner layer of the sac as a result of inflammation from infection or injury

PERICARDITIS

Inflammation of the **pericardium**. The condition features chest pain, fever and disturbed heart action

PERICARDIUM

The outer sac that surrounds the heart

PERNICIOUS ANAEMIA

A type of anaemia caused by vitamin B_{12} deficiency. The red cells are enlarged but the oxygen-carrying capacity of the blood is reduced

PLACEBO

A chemically inert or innocuous substance given in place of a drug either for purposes of research or, in cases where no treatment is necessary, because the patient expects a prescription

PLAQUE

A deposit of fatty material, cholesterol, degenerate muscle cells and fibrous tissue in the inner lining of an **artery** in the condition of **atherosclerosis**

PLEURISY

Inflammation of the double membrane lining the lungs and chest cavity (pleura)

PULMONARY ARTERY

The blood vessel that carries blood from the heart to the lungs

PULMONARY OEDEMA

Excess fluid retention in the lungs

PULMONARY VALVE

The heart valve between the right **ventricle** and the **pulmonary artery**. It has three flaps, or cusps

GLOSSARY

RHEUMATIC FEVER

A disease that causes inflammation in various tissues throughout the body. The main effect on the heart can be a thickening or scarring of the heart's valves, leading to narrowing of and/or leakage through the valves

RIGHT ATRIUM

See **Atrium**

RIGHT VENTRICLE

See **Ventricle**

SICK SINUS-NODE SYNDROME

Abnormal function of the heart's natural pacemaker which leads to a slow or irregular heart rate

SINUS BRADYCARDIA

A slow, regular heart rate caused by reduced electrical activity in the heart's natural pacemaker

SINUS, OR SINOATRIAL (S-A), NODE

The heart's natural pacemaker, which produces the electrical impulses that travel down to reach the ventricular muscle, causing the heart to contract

SPHYGMOMANOMETER

An instrument for measuring blood pressure

STERNUM

The breastbone

STETHOSCOPE

An instrument for listening to sounds within the body

STREPTOKINASE

A drug used to dissolve blood clots. Given in the early stages of a heart attack, it may limit the damage caused to the heart muscle

STRESS TEST

An **electrocardiogram** taken while the patient is undergoing exercise or stress, as on a treadmill. The test evaluates the heart's response to the stress of physical exercise. It is most often performed to determine the cause of unexplained chest pain when coronary heart disease is suspected

SUPERIOR VENA CAVA

One of two very large veins into which all the circulating deoxygenated blood drains; starts at the top of the chest and travels some three inches downwards before connecting to the right **atrium**. It collects blood from the upper trunk, head, neck and arms

SYNCOPE

Fainting, as a result of insufficient blood flow to the brain

SYSTOLE

The peaks of blood pressure measured in the arteries. It occurs when the heart contracts with each heartbeat

TACHYCARDIA

An abnormally fast heartbeat

THROMBOEMBOLISM

The blockage of a blood vessel by a particle that has broken away from a blood clot

THROMBOSIS

The formation or presence of a blood clot inside a blood vessel or cavity of the heart

TISSUE-TYPE PLASMINOGEN ACTIVATOR (TPA)

A genetically engineered enzyme that dissolves blood clots. It is used in the treatment of heart attacks, severe progressive angina pectoris, and blockage of an **artery**

TRICUSPID VALVE

The heart valve between the right **atrium** and the right **ventricle**. It has three flaps, or cusps

TRIGLYCERIDE

A fat that comes from food or is made in the body from other energy sources such as carbohydrates or proteins. Normal body fats are triglycerides

VALVULAR REGURGITATION

A backflow of liquid from valves

VASODILATOR

A drug that causes the muscle in the walls of arteries to relax, allowing the vessel to dilate (widen)

VEIN

A thin-walled blood vessel that returns blood towards the heart from the various organs and tissues of the body

VENTRICLE

One of the two lower chambers of the heart

VENTRICULAR ANEURYSM

A ballooning of a portion of the wall of a ventricle, usually due to the pressure of blood acting on an area weakened by **infarction**

VENTRICULAR FIBRILLATION

A condition in which the ventricles contract in a rapid, fluttering, non-synchronous and uncoordinated fashion so that no blood is pumped from the heart. This is one of the forms of cardiac arrest and must be corrected by defibrillation before normal heart rhythm can be restored. Ventricular fibrillation often happens early in a heart attack

REFERENCES

'ACE inhibitors in heart attack', *New England Journal of Medicine* January 12 1994: 118

'ACE inhibitors and heart attack', *Lancet* 30 July 1994: 279

'Advances in treatment of heart attacks, angina', *British Medical Journal* 19 November 1994: 1343

'Age and cardiovascular system', *Cardiology in Practice* October 1989: 18

'AIDS and heart disease', *Cardiology in Practice* November 1989: 11

'Air bag heart rupture', *New England Journal of Medicine* February 4 1993: 358

'Alcohol and coronary heart disease reduction', *British Medical Journal* 17 July 91

'Alcohol and the heart', *British Journal of Hospital Medicine* 16 November 1994: 497

'Alcohol and heart disease', *British Medical Journal* 27 November 1993: 1373

'Alcohol and heart disease', *Lancet* 13 February 1993: 387

'Alcohol and heart irregularity', *British Medical Journal* 30 May 1992: 1394

'Alcohol and ischaemic heart disease', *British Medical Journal* 7 September 1991: 553, 565

'Alcohol intake and heart disease', *New England Journal of Medicine* December 16 1993: 1829

'Alcohol with a meal reduces heart disease', *British Medical Journal* 16 April 1994: 1003

'Alcohol and skeletal heart muscle', *New England Journal of Medicine* February 16 1989: 409

'Ambulatory oxygen in heart failure', *Lancet* 14 November 1992: 1192

'Amiodarone and heart failure', *New England Journal of Medicine* July 13 1995: 77, 121

'Angina-like pain heart or oesophagus?', *British Journal of Hospital Medicine* June 1990: 443

'Angioplasty for heart attack', *New England Journal of Medicine* March 11 1993: 673 680 685 726

'Artificial heart', *Journal of the American Medical Association* October 1991: 1907

'Artificial hearts', *British Medical Journal* 1 April 1989: 843

'Artificial heart support', *British Journal of Hospital Medicine* May 1989: 420 June 8

'Artificial heart support', *British Journal of Hospital Medicine* June 1989: 520

'Artificial heart valve failure', *British Medical Journal* 22 October 1988: 996

'Artificial heart valve failure', *Lancet* 1 February 1992: 257

'Artificial heart valve life', *British Journal of Hospital Medicine* March 1990: 179

'Aspirin and congenital heart defects', *New England Journal of Medicine* December 14 1989: 1639

'Aspirin dose to prevent heart attack', *Journal of the American Medical Association* November 24 1993: 2502

'Athletes' hearts', *Lancet* 7 November 1992: 1132

'Baldness and heart attacks', *Journal of the American Medical Association* February 24 1993: 998 1035

'Balloon dilatation of heart valves', *British Medical Journal* 29 August 1992: 487

'Barker hypothesis prenatal origin of heart disease', *British Medical Journal* 18 February 1995: 411

'Broken heart how to avoid sudden death', *Journal of the Royal Society of Medicine* August 1993: 438

'Can Chlamydia cause heart disease?', *New Scientist* 18 June 1994: 17

'Captopril and heart attack', *Lancet* 18 March 1995: 686

'Carbon monoxide and coronary heart disease', *New England Journal of Medicine* November 23 1989: 1474

'Cardiac heart denervation physiology', *British Journal of Hospital Medicine* 2 September 1992: 220

'Cardiomyoplasty for heart failure', *British Journal of Hospital Medicine* 7 October 1992: 355

'Cholesterol and coronary heart disease', *British Medical Journal* 4 July 1992: 15

'Cholesterol and coronary heart disease', *Journal of the American Medical Association* February 12 1992: 816

'Cholesterol and heart disease', *Journal of the Royal Society of Medicine* August 1994: 450

'Cholesterol and heart disease', *New England Journal of Medicine* February 4 1993: 313, 321

'Cholesterol and heart disease Doll', *New Scientist* 21 November 1992: 32

'Cholesterol lowering heart disease', *British Medical Journal* 15 May 1993: 1313

'Chronic heart failure', *Lancet* 11 July 1992: 1988 92

'Circadian rhythm and heart attacks', *Journal of the American Medical Association* June 3 1992: 2935

'Coagulation factor V gene and heart attacks', *New England Journal of Medicine* April 6 1995: 912

'Cocaine childbirth heart attacks', *New Scientist* 18 December 1993: 15

'Coffee cholesterol heart disease', *British Medical Journal* 6 April 1991: 804

'Coffee consumption and coronary heart disease', *British Medical Journal* 3 March 1990: 566

'Congenital heart defects', *British Journal of Hospital Medicine* 3 November 1993: 513 523

'Controlling chaos in the heart chaos' *Science* 28 August 1992: 1230

'Coronary disease in heart transplants', *Lancet* 19 December 1992: 1500

'Coronary heart disease cholesterol elderly', *British Medical Journal* 13 July 1991: 69

'Coronary heart disease populations low cholesterol', *British Medical Journal* 3 August 91

'Coronary heart disease in Scotland', *Lancet* 11 August 1990: 349

'Coronary heart disease what do we know?', *Cardiology in Practice* November 1989: 20, 28

'Cutting aberrant heart conduction pathways', *Lancet* 29 June

'Depression and heart disease', *Lancet* 4 September 1993: 570

'Diabetes and ischaemic heart disease', *Journal of the American Medical Association* February 5 1991: 627

'Drug aspirin in ischaemic heart disease', *New England Journal of Medicine* November 12 1992: 1455

'Drug aspirin ischaemic heart disease review', *New England Journal of Medicine* July 16 1992: 175

'Drugs of abuse and heart attack', *Lancet* 31 October 1992: 1069

'Early ECG evidence heart attack thrombolysis', *British Medical Journal* 14 August 1993: 409

'Education and heart attacks in India', *British Medical Journal* 19 November 1994: 1332

'Emotion stress and the heart', *Cardiology in Practice* June 1989: 11

'Endstage heart failure; surgical options', *British Journal of Hospital Medicine* 3 May 1995: 428, 435

'Exercise and coronary heart disease', *New England Journal of Medicine* June 24 1993: 1852

'Fats and heart disease', *Lancet* 28 June 1994: 1518 1528

'Fatty acids and heart disease', *Lancet* 6 March 1993: 581

'Fetal heart transplant ethics', *Journal of the American Medical Association* January 20 1993: 401

'Fetal nutrition adult heart disease', *Lancet* 10 April 1993: 938

'Fetal origins of coronary heart disease', *British Medical Journal* 15 July 1995: 171

'Fish oil and the heart', *Lancet* 16 December 1989: 1450

'Fish oil and heart attacks', *New England Journal of Medicine* April 13 1995: 977, 1024

'Fish oil and heart disease', *Lancet* 30 September 1989: 757

REFERENCES

'Fish oil and heart disease', *British Medical Journal* 1 April 1995: 819

'Free radicals antioxidants heart attack', *Lancet* 4 December 1993: 1379

'Free radicals and heart attack', *Lancet* 17 April 1993: 990

'Free radicals heart disease vit E', *New England Journal of Medicine* May 20 1993: 1444 1487

'Free radicals vitamin E heart disease', *New England Journal of Medicine* November 4 1993: 1426

'French paradox wine, diet, antioxidants coronary heart disease', *Lancet* 24 December 1994: 1719

'Genes therapy for heart failure', *New England Journal of Medicine* March 23 1995: 817

'Genetics and heart disease', *Lancet* 17 April 1993: 995

'German heart valve scandal', *British Medical Journal* 6 May 1995: 1160

'Glucose fatty acids and heart attack', *Lancet* 15 January 1994: 155

'Green tea protective against heart and liver disease?', *British Medical Journal* 18 March 1995: 693

'Heart arrhythmias', *Cardiology in Practice* August 1989: 26

'Heart arrhythmias', *Journal of the Royal Society of Medicine* February 1994: 67

'Heart attack management', *British Medical Journal* 29 October 1994: 1129

'Heart attacks', *New Scientist* Inside science No 62

'Heart attacks and exertion', *New England Journal of Medicine* December 2 1993: 1677

'Heart attack after surgery', *British Medical Journal* 13 May 1995: 1215

'Heart attack in women', *British Medical Journal* 3 September 1994: 563

'Heart catheter ablation conduction problems', *Journal of the American Medical Association* October 21 1992: 2091

'Heart disease, anticipating', *New Scientist* 2 September 1989

'Heart disease black and white compared', *New England Journal of Medicine* August 26 1993: 600

'Heart disease and early deprivation', *Lancet* 6 June 1992: 1386

'Heart disease fish oil', *Cardiology in Practice* March 1990: 26

'Heart disease in AIDS', *British Journal of Sexual Medicine* April 1990: 111

'Heart disease screening waste of time?', *British Medical Journal* 29 January 1994: 285

'Heart disease and sex', *British Journal of Sexual Medicine* January 1989: 25

'Heart disease starts in childhood', *British Medical Journal* 28 March 1992: 789

'Heart disease why less in France', *British Medical Journal* 17 December 1988: 1559

'Heart failure', *British Journal of Hospital Medicine* 21 June 1995: 43

'Heart failure adrenaline receptor gene', *New Scientist* 14 May 1994: 16

'Heart failure cardiomyoplasty use of latissimus dorsi muscle', *British Medical Journal* 8 June 91: 1353

'Heart failure cardiomyoplasty latissimus dorsi', *Lancet* 8 June 91: 1383

'Heart failure diagnosis management', *British Medical Journal* 29 January 1994: 321

'Heart failure management', *British Journal of Hospital Medicine* 9 January 1992: 16

'Heart failure treatment', *Advanced Medicine*: 243

'Heart failure treatment', *British Medical Journal* 14 December 1994: 1631

'Heart failure treatment', *British Medical Journal* 9 July 1988: 83

'Heart and heart-lung transplant', *Lancet* 12 May 1990: 1126

'Heart in hypertension review', *New England Journal of Medicine* October 1 1992: 998

'Heart and lung transplant', *British Medical Journal* 1 August 87

'Heart lung transplant results', *Lancet* 27 June 1992: 1583

'Heart monitoring of fetuses fetal distress', *New Scientist* 2 February 1991: 38

'Heart transplant follow-up', *British Medical Journal* 9 January 1993: 98

'Heart transplantation', *British Medical Journal* 15 April 1989: 979

'Heart transplantation, current state', *British Journal of Hospital Medicine* April 1987: 37

'Heart transplantation – the next decade', *British Journal of Hospital Medicine* 3 May 1995: 440

'Heart transplantation – status', *New England Journal of Medicine* December 1986: 1577

'Heart valves which are best?', *Lancet* 3 November 1990: 1115

'HRT and heart attacks', *New England Journal of Medicine* April 15 1993: 1069 1115

'Hyperventilation and the heart', *Cardiology in Practice* September 1989: 20

'Immunity and heart disease', *New England Journal of Medicine* April 21 1994: 1129

'IV magnesium sulphate for heart attack', *Lancet* 27 June 1992: 1553

'Lifestyle and reversing coronary heart disease', *Lancet* 21 July 1990: 129

'Linolenic fish oil heart disease', *Lancet* 11 June 1994: 1443

'Lipoproteins and heart disease', *Scientific American* June 1992: 26

'Lipoproteins heart disease', *Journal of the American Medical Association* November 10 1993: 2195

'Living alone after heart attack', *Journal of the American Medical Association* January 22 1992: 515

'Low birth weight and heart disease', *Lancet* 29 January 1994: 260

'Low tar cigarettes smoking heart risk', *British Medical Journal* 12 June 1993: 1567

'Magnesium and the heart' *Sci & Med* May 1995: 28

'Magnesium and heart attack', *Lancet* 2 April 1994: 807

'Magnesium in heart attacks', *British Medical Journal* 25 March 1995: 751

'Malaria transmitted heart transplant', *British Medical Journal* 14 December 91

'Mechanical heart support', *Cardiology in Practice* January 1990: 20

'Mechanical v biological heart valves', *New England Journal of Medicine* May 6 1993: 1289

'Melatonin in coronary heart disease', *Lancet* 3 June 1995: 1408

'Milk butter and heart disease', *Lancet* 9 March 1991: 607 1442

'Mortality from heart disease in inter-regional migrants', *British Medical Journal* 18 February 1995: 423

'MRI of the heart', *British Journal of Hospital Medicine* 20 January 1993: 90

'Murder of Victor Chang heart surgeon', *British Medical Journal* 21–28 December 1991: 1583

'Nitric oxide and heart failure', *Lancet* 6 August 1994: 371

'Obesity and coronary heart disease in women', *New England Journal of Medicine* March 29 1990: 928

'Oestrogen heart protection', *Lancet* 15 May 1993: 1264

'Passive smoking and heart disease', *British Medical Journal* 15 December 1990: 1343

'Passive smoking and heart disease', *Journal of the American Medical Association* January 1 1992: 94

'Pets and heart disease health', *New Scientist* 9 October 1993: 30

'Physical activity risk of heart attack', *New England Journal of Medicine* June 2 1994: 1549

'Portable heart assist pump', *Journal of the American Medical Association* November 20 1991: 2666

'Predicting heart attack outcome', *Lancet* 3 April 1993: 855

'Preventing coronary heart disease in women', *New England Journal of Medicine* June 29 1995: 1758

'Prevention of heart failure', *New England Journal of Medicine* September 3 1992: 725

'Prosthetic heart valve failures', *Lancet* 1 January 1993: 9

'Renin and heart disease', *New England Journal of Medicine* August 26 1993: 616

'Reperfusion injury after heart attack free radicals', *British Medical Journal* 25 February 1995: 477

'Reuse of a transplanted heart', *New England Journal of Medicine* February 4 1993: 319

'Review of heart surgery', *Journal of the American Medical Association* July 15 1992

'Risk of heart attack during TIAs', *Lancet* 12 September 1992: 630

'Scottish hospital death rates from heart attacks', *British Medical Journal* 14 December 1994: 1599

'Sex and heart attacks', *New Scientist* 8 January 1994: 13

'Skeletal muscle in heart failure', *Lancet* 5 December 1992: 1383

'Sleep and heart attacks', *New England Journal of Medicine* February 4 1993: 303

'Stress does not cause heart disease', *New Scientist* 12 August 1995: 9

'Thrombolysis in heart attack', *British Journal of Hospital Medicine* 7 June 1995: 575

'Thrombolysis after heart attacks', *British Medical Journal* 22 January 1994: 216

'Thyrotoxicosis and the heart', *New England Journal of Medicine* July 9 1992: 94

'Tissue-engineered heart valves', *Scientific American* June 1995: 24

'Tobacco snuff and heart attacks', *British Medical Journal* 21 November 1992: 1252

'Trans fatty acids and heart disease', *Lancet* 4 February 1995: 269

'Twins and heart disease', *New England Journal of Medicine* April 14 1994: 1041

'Walnuts heart disease and blood pressure', *New England Journal of Medicine* March 4 1993: 593

'Warm heart surgery', *Lancet* 4 April 1992: 841

'Westernised Asians and heart disease', *Lancet* 18 February 1995: 401

'Which heart valve?', *Lancet* 23 March 1991: 705

'Wine and coronary heart disease', *Lancet* 1 August 1992: 313

'Wine and heart disease', *Lancet* 20 June 1992: 1523

'Wine and mortality from heart attacks and stroke', *British Medical Journal* 6 May 1995: 1165

'Women and coronary heart disease', *British Medical Journal* 1 May 1993: 1145

INDEX

BLOOD PRESSURE: QUESTIONS YOU HAVE...ANSWERS YOU NEED

Karla Morales

High blood pressure – hypertension – is one of the most common and most serious of all health conditions.

This vital guide cuts through the medical jargon and clearly answers the most commonly asked questions about high blood pressure, including invaluable advice about how to prevent, and cope with, the disease:

- What causes high blood pressure?
- Can high blood pressure be cured?
- Is it safe to exercise?
- What are the dangers of low blood pressure?
- How does diet affect blood pressure?
- What drugs are used for treatment and how do they work?

PROSTATE: QUESTIONS YOU HAVE...ANSWERS YOU NEED

Sandra Salmans

Most men experience prostate problems at some stage in their life. Yet there are many myths and misunderstandings about the prostate gland.

This clear, practical guide cuts through the medical jargon and answers hundreds of questions including invaluable advice about the range of treatments available for prostatitis, benign enlargement of the prostate and prostate cancer.

- What goes wrong with the prostate?
- What are the symptoms?
- What drugs and surgical treatments are available?
- Is benign prostatic hyperplasia (BPH) an inevitable part of the ageing process?
- Does treatment for prostatic disease necessarily result in impotency?

BLOOD PRESSURE: QUESTIONS YOU HAVE…
ANSWERS YOU NEED   0 7225 3314 4   £3.99   ☐

PROSTATE: QUESTIONS YOU HAVE…
ANSWERS YOU NEED   0 7225 3420 5   £3.99   ☐

All these books are available from your local bookseller or can be
ordered direct from the publishers.

To order direct just tick the titles you want and fill in the form below:

Name: _____

_____

Address: _____

_____

_____

Postcode: _____

Send to Thorsons Mail Order, Dept 3, HarperCollins*Publishers*,
Westerhill Road, Bishopbriggs, Glasgow G64 2QT.
Please enclose a cheque or postal order or your authority to debit
your Visa/Access account —

Credit card no: _____

_____

Expiry date: _____

_____

Signature: _____

— up to the value of the cover price plus:
UK & BFPO: Add £1.00 for the first book and 25p for each additional
book ordered.
Overseas orders including Eire: Please add £2.95 service charge.
Books will be sent by surface mail but quotes for airmail dispatches
will be given on request.

24-HOUR TELEPHONE ORDERING SERVICE FOR ACCESS/VISA
CARDHOLDERS — TEL: 0141 772 2281.